LOURDES LIBRARY
GWYNEDD-MERCY COLLEGE
GWYNEDD VALLEY, PA. 19437

AF179515

LOURDES LIBRARY
GWYNEDD-MERCY COLLEGE
GWYNEDD VALLEY, PA. 19437

THE HISTORY OF AMERICAN NURSING

Edited by
Susan Reverby, Wellesley College

LOURDES LIBRARY
GWYNEDD-MERCY COLLEGE
GWYNEDD VALLEY, PA. 19437

A GARLAND SERIES

LOURDES LIBRARY
GWYNEDD-MERCY COLLEGE
GWYNEDD VALLEY, PA. 19437

RG
962.5
.N4
C367
1984

FOLKS DO GET BORN

LOURDES LIBRARY
GWYNEDD-MERCY COLLEGE
GWYNEDD VALLEY, PA 19437

Marie Campbell

LOURDES LIBRARY
GWYNEDD-MERCY COLLEGE
GWYNEDD VALLEY, PA 19437

84578

GARLAND PUBLISHING, INC.
NEW YORK • LONDON
1984

For a complete list of the titles in this series see the final pages of this volume.

Copyright 1946, © 1974 by Marie Campbell.
This edition is published by arrangement with Holt, Rinehart and Winston.

This facsimile has been made from a copy in the Beinecke Library of Yale University.

Library of Congress Cataloging in Publication Data

Campbell, Marie, 1907–
Folks do get born.

(The History of American nursing)
Reprint. Originally published: New York : Rinehart, c1946.
1. Midwives—Georgia—History. 2. Afro-American nurses—Georgia—History. I. Title. II. Series.
RG961.G4C36 1984 362.1'982 83-49143
ISBN 0-8240-6504-2 (alk. paper)

The volumes in this series are printed on acid-free, 250-year-life paper.

Printed in the United States of America

Folks Do Get Born

By Marie Campbell

CLOUD WALKING

FOLKS DO GET BORN

Folks Do Get Born

MARIE CAMPBELL

Illustrated by Clare Leighton

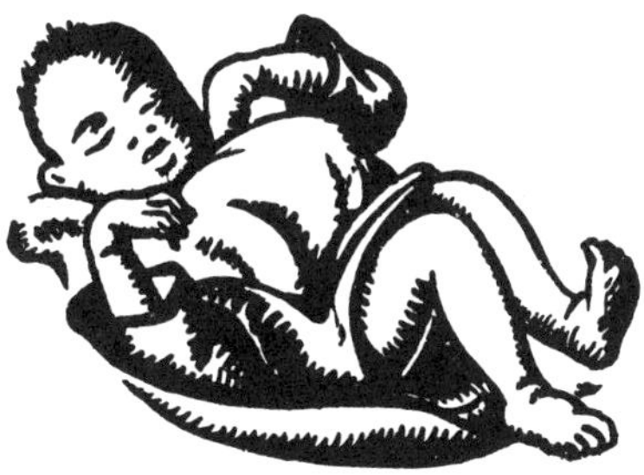

RINEHART & COMPANY,
Incorporated
New York Toronto

PUBLISHER'S NOTE

Readers in America unanimously approved the size of books produced during the war because they were lighter in weight and more economical in shelf space. We are therefore continuing to issue our books, complete and unabridged, in these popular sizes.

COPYRIGHT, 1946, BY MARIE CAMPBELL
PRINTED IN THE UNITED STATES OF AMERICA
BY J. J. LITTLE AND IVES COMPANY, NEW YORK
ALL RIGHTS RESERVED

For

AUNT JEANIE *and* MAM BOB

LOURDES LIBRARY
GWYNEDD-MERCY COLLEGE
GWYNEDD VALLEY, PA 19437

Acknowledgments

The public health nurses who have helped with this book have generously asked to be left in the background because they feel the book belongs to the granny-midwives. But without the help of these nurses the book could not have been written, and I want to recognize their services. Specifically, I wish to thank the following nurses:

Mrs. Abbie R. Weaver, Director of Public Health Nursing for the State of Georgia, Miss Vera A. Mingledorff, Mrs. Ethel H. Ham, Miss Fannielu McWhorter, Mrs. Palestine P. Coleman, Miss Margaret Gardner, Miss Lucia Massee, Miss Nell Clark, Mrs. Anne H. Dobbins, Mrs. Bessie F. Swan, Mrs. Anna Brown, Miss Josephine Kinman, Miss Lula Smith, Miss Jewel Page, Lieutenant Helen P. Caldwell A.N.C., Miss Girtha Ree Wilkerson, Miss Alice Battle, Miss Claudia Marie Durham, Mrs. Beatrice J. Trammell, Miss Margaret W. Thomas, Mrs. Josephine P. Batton, Miss Pearl C. Motley, and Miss Elsie Crosby.

Also I should like to acknowledge permission from the editors of *Public Health Nursing* and of *Georgia's Health* to quote from articles published in those magazines, and from Brandt & Brandt to quote from "Prayer" by Stephen Vincent Benét. I am grateful to Miss Laura Blackburn for allowing me to use parts of her article in *Public Health Nursing*.

And I would not forget to mention my gratitude to my student-typists, Juanita Estes and Dixie Grimsley.

Contents

PART I

PART II

Part One

In the Manner of Explaining

THE material in this book has come largely from the midwives, and its arrangement has been a matter of discussion in one of their groups. After they had deliberated long and seriously, their chairman on their behalf gave this advice: "We think you better put first the part that is in the manner of explaining. That's the part that tells about the granny-midwives being on the Board, about their connections with the nurses, about their midwife clubs and their other kinds of meetings, and all kinds of true facts about the grannies. Then when folks read the part of your book where the granny-midwives talk sociable in a kind of story fashion, then folks will have in the back of their minds the part that is in the manner of explaining, and they will know and understand all of what the grannies are talking about and not be ignorant."

Just by way of explaining, the terms *midwife, granny-midwife,* and *granny,* used interchangeably in this book, all refer to the traditional colored midwife as she is known in rural Georgia. Except in a few mountainous counties in the northeastern section of the state, the midwives in Georgia—as in other states of the lower South—are largely colored women, usually women past middle age. More specifically, the midwives in this book are Negro women in rural Georgia counties which have a high percentage of Negro population. It is in such counties that the midwives are most numerous.

The nurses mentioned here are public health nurses doing field work in Georgia counties where supervising midwives is part of their work. Most of these nurses are white women, a few are colored. As to their part in this book, they said, "Consider us merely incidental to your knowing the granny-midwives. This book definitely belongs to them."

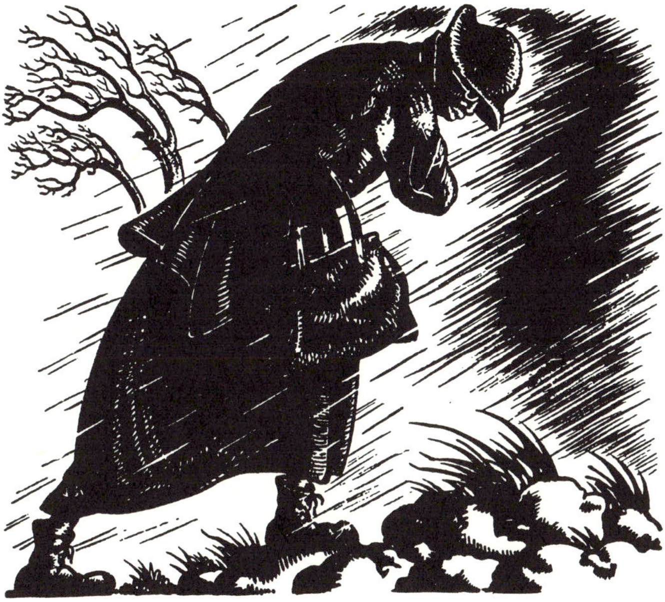

I Got a Heap to Do at Once

THERE is indeed "a heap to do at once" for the granny-midwives who usher into the world 26 per cent of all the babies born in Georgia. Only a decade ago it was 42 per cent. These grannies do not realize that they are the "midwife problem." They know simply that somebody has to attend at a birthing, and that there have never been enough doctors to go around. So through the years they have done what they could.

If you were to ask almost any Georgia midwife about the practice of midwifery through the years, she would take you back to Bible times. To try to look back beyond the Bible is outside her imagining. She would cite you the first chapter of Exodus, where the increase in population among the Hebrews in Egypt had become so rapid and so great that the King of Egypt decided he would have to use drastic measures to limit the Hebrew population in his country. So he called to him two of the Hebrew midwives and ordered that all male children born to Hebrew mothers be killed at birth by the midwives. Our present day colored midwives think there must have been a large number of these Hebrew grannies, "for two women couldn't catch enough babies every year to get the King of the Country worried about how many." Of one thing they are certain: these Hebrew midwives were God-fearing women who disobeyed the King of Egypt and let the boy babies among the Hebrews live. Our midwives claim that their own strong religious strain regarding their profession "reaches back to them granny-midwives in the Bible."

The granny-midwife in Georgia would tell you—and rightly so—that the colored midwife came into Georgia with the coming of slavery. One old midwife claims a tradition of midwifery being practiced by women in her family "all the way straight back" to their tribe in Africa where some midwife ancestor of hers was captured and sold into slavery. She brought the practice of her profession with her to America, handing it down to some close female relative, usually a daughter, in each succeeding generation. This old colored woman who is the last of this long family line of midwives grieves because the family tradition ends with her. "I just ain't been able to persuade none of the young women in my family to learn to catch babies," she says. "They don't feel called to do work that carries them out across the country at all times of the day or night and in all kinds of weather, good or bad. And they want to do work with more regular hours and with better pay. So I reckon I'm the last to be a granny-midwife in my family."

What she says of a long line of women practicing midwifery in her family may very well be true. It is historically true that in slavery days certain of the older and more intelligent Negro women were delegated to attend the women in the quarters in childbirth. Sometimes their services were extended to the care of women in the household of the plantation owners. Letters, entries in diaries, and other such records indicate that the family doctor of the landowner was sometimes called upon to instruct the midwife in obstetrical procedures. Sometimes she learned incidentally from the doctor simply by being with him on a case without any prearranged plan that he was to teach her. All too many antebellum midwives learned all they knew from another midwife, usually an older relative, under whose wing they entered the profession. Many customs and superstitions were handed down, some of them dangerous to the lives of mothers and babies.

After freedom the situation was not appreciably changed. The midwife was increasingly called upon by women of either color who could not afford or were unable to secure the services of a doctor in childbirth. Many midwives continued to have no training other than what was passed on to them from other midwives. Some learned what they could from being on cases with doctors. For generations very little attention was paid to the midwife and her procedures and standards of practice.

"It's just the last twenty years that the granny-midwives have been on the Board," explained Aunt Dilly, a retired midwife. "Before that time we never had no connection with the Board of Health in this state. We never had no caps and masks and hospital gowns to wear, nor no nurses training us how to tend on a woman in childbed according to the New Law. I caught babies by the Old Law and then by the New Law, and I can recollect plain when us grannies was first told that according to the New Law we was forbid to catch babies without we had a license blank and was on the Board. Whatever the Law, we have aimed to be faithful, but they ain't so many of us no more as there used to be."

When in 1925 the State Board of Health first assumed responsibility for supervising and licensing midwives, there were approximately 9,000 granny-midwives practicing in Georgia. In 1944 the number had decreased to 2,200. Comparatively few candidates for midwifery have appeared in the last few years. So Mam Bob's statement that grannies will some day be "a nigh-gone thing" is by no means farfetched. This decrease in the number of midwives indicates an urgent need to replace them with better maternity service. This need is particularly urgent in rural areas where doctors are so few. Some communities are now without the services of either a doctor or a midwife. This means that neighbors or members of the family have to care for mothers in childbirth. As one old granny-midwife says, "They are in a tight corner when they can't have not even a midwife there with a woman in her misery." Another midwife at her retirement petitioned the Almighty to "give folks the minds to know and the strength to do, so they can manage for better ways of looking after their women folks when they birth their babies."

Aunt Jeanie did not know that in a mountainous corner of Northeast Georgia a whole county had already put their minds and their strength together "to manage better ways of looking after" their mothers and babies. The result of their coöperative thinking and doing is the Rabun County Maternity Hospital for the use of *all* their mothers regardless of their ability or inability to pay. This Maternity Hospital serves a county that is entirely rural and largely mountainous. Except for the small town of Clayton, the population is largely scattered. The Rabun County Maternity Hospital, opened November 20, 1942, represents a real bit of pioneering on the part of Rabun County's forward looking citizens, for it is one of the very first of its kind in the rural South. Other such maternity shelters are planned for rural areas after the war when medical, nursing, and housekeeping staffs will be available.

For the past few years—and it is only the past few years that there have been such schools in the United

States—the Georgia Department of Public Health has been sending public health nurses for six months' training in midwifery at Maternity Center in New York City, at Frontier Graduate School in Midwifery in connection with the Frontier Nursing Service at Wendover, Kentucky, and at Tuskegee School for Training Nurses in Midwifery at Tuskegee, Alabama. As yet nurse-midwives are few in number in the United States and few in Georgia. The midwifery schools in this country can take only a few students each year, and at present most public health nurses are too busy to be released for training.

The school which trains colored nurses in midwifery at Tuskegee is an outgrowth of joint thinking on the part of public health people throughout the South in relation to the high infant and maternal mortality and lack of medical facilities. The problem was discussed with the Children's Bureau, Maternity Center Association, and other leaders in the field. The Tuskegee School for Training Nurses in Midwifery, opened in September 1941, resulted from this planning. Most of its students come from the public health departments of Southern states.

Training public health nurses in midwifery and opening rural maternity hospitals such as the one in Rabun County are evidences that plans for better maternity service to reach out into the farthest rural districts are beginning to become reality. But it is well to keep in mind that some communities are without either the services of a physician or a midwife. It is well to remember that if the granny-midwives were not allowed to practice at all, there is—and this is especially true of rural sections—no one as yet to take their place.

"Us granny-midwives have got a heap to do yet," they say. "We just hope we can hold out faithful till there get to be hospitals and doctors and nurses in plenty for everybody, even for them that can't pay no price big enough to count for much. But that time ain't come yet, so us grannies still catch a lots of babies with nobody to look to for help but the Lord and the health nurse. They both got right long patience with us, considering they both got a heap to do and troubles a-plenty of their own."

The public health nurses in Georgia—and Georgia's midwife problem is little different from that in many Southern states—spend much time and effort in endeavoring to train and instruct the grannies in sanitary care of mothers and babies. The midwives' expressions become as familiar to the nurses as their own, and they can and do converse easily in the midwife's own language. This ability stands the nurse in good stead in interpreting correspondence from her midwives, for many a midwife's lack of formal education forces her to resort to phonetic spelling. Nevertheless she has a way of making herself and her wants clearly understood to her nurse. The following letter was received by a public health nurse from a granny-midwife and the drawings as shown on the reproduction of the original are the granny's own. The midwife sketched is a self-portrait.

So to say good morning to you. Pleas i want you to make me out a Lison Blank for grannie doctor. Thay is a tight cornder out here. Need us right now. Say thay ant noBody clost anuff. Want me. i want you to fix me up. i Bee up just as soon as i can get a way to come. it 10 miles out here an no way to get to town now tell i can catch a way.

i has moved with Mr. Felton Rice, R 2 — 10 miles. Lison Blank, how can i get one. can you fix me up. i got to get to work some where that i am aBle to do. so i can do that medwife grannie. i want my JoB Back. i was tort to Be a grannie Like this. . . . Cisus cut to inch tie to inch. thay need me now. see i Ben tort By clinic nurce to Pashon to shew them just what to do for them self an what to yose to keep comfort a while. i am ready to heare—yes, you can get it fix up. this is a needed time out here. 4 (women) i no is gota have me soon as you give me the paper so thay no i am on Board. Put my sine name on Clinic Board for catchin BaBy grannie. it wont Be long Before one go in, she is clost at hand now. i Ben talkin to her tellin her what to do for herself an show her how to fix her Pices on her Bed Like this Put a Pad of Papa an close togeather and sowe it so it wont tar to peaces. i noes what to do how i Bean traned an to fix things the way i Bean showin. Fix me up a order of Books. i am gettin the money (from the patient). Just as soone as you say the Licon is fix up for me to start to work. thay need me now at once. i am talkin to them, shew them what to do. i am getting along good, along the Best as i ExPex to so far an hop to contingen on. i am tryin do for myself for my children got to take care there self. Pleas fix me up a order a Licon Blank an Books to how and what thay do like this . . . fix me up at once. Let me go. i got a heap to do at once. R 2, Mr felton rice Place. he help me.

J

January 11-1944 as to
say good morning if
you pleas i want you to
make me out a lison.
Blank. for grannie doctor
he is a tight cornder out
here need us right now
say that ant no Body
Clost anuff want me i
want you to fix me.
us i Bee up just as
soon as i can get
a way to come it 10
miles out here an no
way to get to town
now till i can catch a
way mrs Sandr health
Clinic Ethes fu Coger i
sas maned with mr
Felton rice R 2 - 10 miles

(2)

Lison Blank how can i
get one can you fix me
up i got get to work
some where. that i am
able to do as i can do
that. med wife granni
i want my JoB Back
i was tort to Be a granni
like this

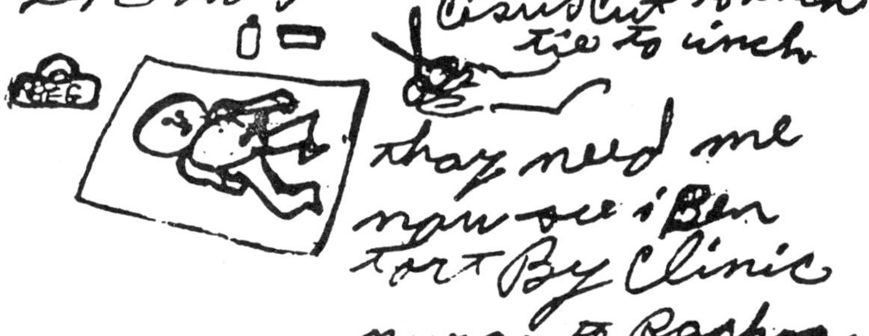

thay need me
now see i Ben
tort By Clinic
nurce to Rashon
to show them
Oust what to do
for them self an what to
yose to keep comfort a
while i am rady to here

3

i noes what to do how i
an Bean traned an to
fix thing the way i Bean
showin. Fix me up a
order of Books i an
gtum the money Just
as soone as you say
the Licon is fix up for
me to start to work
thay need me now
at once i am talkin to
them shew them what
to do i am gettin along
good along the Best as
i Ex Rex to so for. an
sop to Contingen on
i am. tryin to for my
self for my Childrun got
to take Care there self
pleas fix me up a order

Yes you. Can get it
fix up. this is a needed
time for here it it i ng is
got hake me soon as
you give me the Paper
so that ng i am on
Board Put my ~~line~~

name on Clinic Board for
Catchin Baby grannie
it [illegible] Be long Before
one go in she is close
at hand now i Ben talkin
to her tellin her what to
do for her self an show
her how to fix her pieces
on her Bed her Bed like this

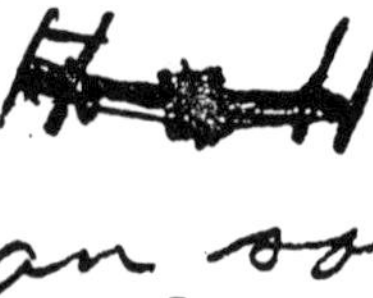

put a pad of Papa
an close to geather
an sore it so it wont tar
to peaces. deadno Line Jos

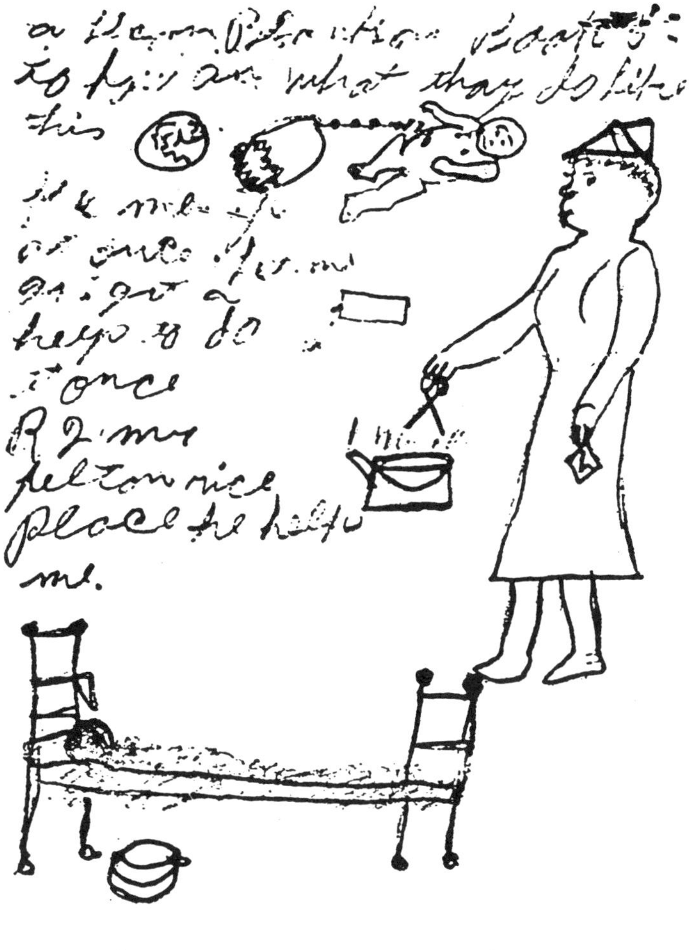
what thay do like
this
once
mr
felton nice
place he help
me.

For those not familiar with the midwife's terminology a glossary of definitions is here offered in the order in which the words occur in the letter.

Lison blank—midwife certificate
Granny doctor—midwife
Clost anuff—close enough
cornder—corner
Midwife grannie—midwife
Tort—taught
Grannie—midwife
Cisus—scissors
Beg—midwife bag
Pashon—patient
Yose—use
Comfort—comfortable
Sine name—full name
Catchin baby—delivering baby
Pices—paper pads
Papa—paper
Tar—tear
Books—Midwife instruction books
Expex—expect
Contingen on—Continue

The "lison blank" which she pleads for so earnestly is the midwife certificate issued annually by the Georgia Department of Public Health to those midwives who regularly attend the public health nurse's classes and are approved for practice in the state. Only the better ones are recommended for the "lison blank," without which they are forbidden to practice.

The "books" which the midwife mentions in her letter are a maternity pamphlet and a booklet of midwife regulations issued by the State Department of of Public Health, stating what the midwife is to do and what not to do. In the booklet these regulations are given in some detail. In their simplest terms the requirements for a midwife, if she is to get and keep her annual "lison blank," are quoted from a granny who has practiced for many years.

"There are things you got to *be*," she says. "You got to be of good moral character, and in your right mind, and you got to be without any disease anybody could catch from you. Another thing is you got to be clean in a personal way and clean in the way you work.

"Then certain things you got to *have*. You got to have a new midwife license every year, and be ready and willing to show it to any person that wants to see. Then you got to have a midwife bag with all the things in it you are supposed to use catching babies and keep your bag clean of germs and ready to be searched any time so the health people can see if they are satisfied with what you got in your midwife bag.

"Then certain things you got to *do*. You can't have no midwife license without you take a blood test every year to see if your blood is moral and you ain't got no bad disease. You got to get a scar from vaccination if you ain't had smallpox. Certain things you are bound by law to do about the mother and the baby. You got to make out birth blanks for the baby, and use eye drops in the baby's eyes, and report to the nurse if the baby's eyes get red. And you are bound to call a doctor if it's too bad a case for you to manage and not take the risk on your own shoulders. Not *one* of them things you got to see to, but every blessed one."

If the midwife violates these regulations, her certificate is taken from her, or, if it is near licensing time, the certificate is not renewed. In either case she is forbidden to continue practicing. She does not accept this deprivation without protest and vigorous efforts to get back in good standing. The foregoing letter is evidence of such efforts. Sometimes she writes only a postcard, of which this communication to the State Health Department from a midwife whose certificate was not renewed is a sample:

> Juest a card. I am willin to obay the rules and Change. I will suggest and see the nurse. I am Willin to Abid. I am sorry I did rong. I will not do so no more long as I live. Your truly.

She did "suggest and see the nurse." In talking about the unsuccessful interview, she said, "The nurse had short patience with me. But she did give me a long private sitting right when she had a heap to do at once. She had a stack of papers to work on high as she was. And it was on a Saturday when my midwife club was meeting and they had to wait for the nurse so they could enter into business."

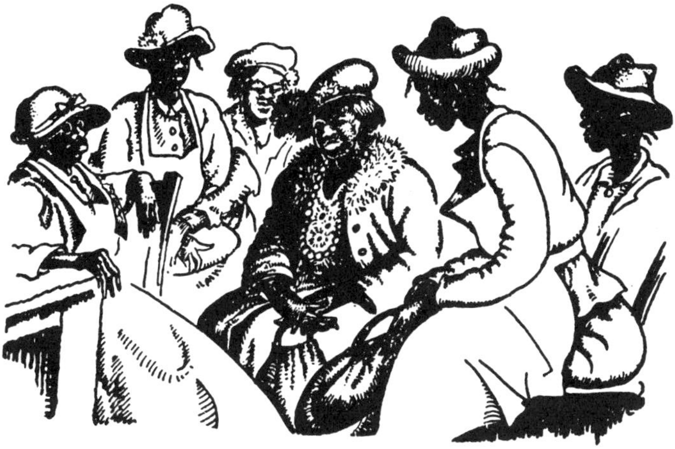

Entered into Business

"IN GEORGIA folks come to town on Saturday, so that's the day our nurses have their meetings every month with the granny-midwives," some of the grannies waiting for their meeting explained. "On Saturday, with so many folks coming to town, we can catch a ride with our colored neighbors or our white connections easier than any other time. Even if we got our own convenience to ride in, Saturday is the best day, for then it is more sociable in town. After the meeting we can do our little trading in the stores and then walk slow around the square and look at the folks and the sights of the town, or gather with our friends and talk, or listen to a street preacher till we get wore out with his gospel shouting."

The nurse sends out post cards, giving notice of time and place of meeting to remind her midwives. In counties which have a special building for the health center, the meetings are held there. Otherwise the meeting place is at the courthouse or at a Negro church. The meetings are usually, though not always, held at the county seat. In a large county, meetings may be held on successive Saturdays at various points most convenient for midwives to reach. When asked about attendance, the midwives said, "Considering that ain't none of us young women, we attends mighty good. We don't want to miss no meetings. When our Midwife Club meets is the only chance we have to talk things over with ourselves and our nurses and thrash out our business, and get whatever help and new learning the nurse can give to us. If bad weather or poor health or catching a baby keeps us from the meeting, our whole heart and mind is to be there. Mostly we writes our nurse a message if we can't come."

This card is a sample of a message to the nurse from a midwife who must be absent but whose "whole heart and mine is to be there."

Ashland Ga

Dear miss massie i am Very sory to tell you that will not get there But my Hole heart an mine is to come if i Dont get there it will all most kill me if I Dont come you no that same mater with me work hard try to get me way to come.

Once in a great while an emergency comes up which at the last minute prevents the nurse from getting to the meeting of her midwives. Then the president of the club takes charge and they carry on as best they can without the nurse. The following is a report on such a meeting conducted in the nurse's absence:

> Preston Ga Aug the 18 1939
> dear miss massie we meet our meeting and the Presdent took charg of the meeting and exyaman the bags and was ok lula sakes came up to the quiement of the laws of the State from eliza koll Preston Ga.

The midwives drift in to the meeting place as they get to town, some early, a few, perhaps, late, though the nurses say those living right in town are more likely to be late. They visit with one another, compare notes on cases, talk of mutual acquaintances, of trips they've taken, of the war, the weather, anything that comes up. The nurse may be busy in her office with catching up on records after a full week of clinics and field work. She may be closeted for a "private sitting" with some midwife who wants to tell her troubles or discuss her problems alone with the nurse. Or the nurse may join the midwives for a sociable chat before time for their meeting to begin. Sometimes a little sociability goes a long way toward creating or sustaining good will and a spirit of coöperation.

The meeting is presided over by the president of the club who says, "The meeting will now be in order, and we'll look to the Lord and then enter into business." The midwives are very religious and their meetings of whatever kind begin with a devotional which "looks to the Lord." Singing comes first. They love to sing and sometimes it is hard to stop them. Nurses say that recently a few midwives have a tendency to want to sing gospel hymns, but almost always the songs are the old spirituals which the nurses and the midwives like best, such as: "Down by the Riverside," "I Shall Not Be Moved," "When the Saints Come Marching In," "Standing in the Need of Prayer." The last mentioned can be sung indefinitely with variations on the relatives.

Bible reading or repeating Bible verses follows the singing. A nurse tells of her first midwife meeting, when she hesitated, not knowing whether or not she too was expected to repeat a Bible verse. One of the oldest midwives spoke up with, "I'll say a verse for the white lady"—and repeated "Thou shalt not steal."

The devotional closes with prayers which are fervent and vivid petitions to the Almighty. The nurse is prayed for at length and in the most graphic terms. "Hold up her hands in strength for the work You got for her to do. Keep her in her right mind at all times and more specially when things go wrong. Make in her a warm heart for folks different from her and not so good as her. Give her a long patience with us granny-midwives. Dear Lord, prop up our nurse on every weak and leaning side. . . ." The prayers are accompanied by comments of emphasis and approval. Sometimes a song starts, which threatens to drown out the prayer but never does completely.

The religious part of the meeting over, the president

says, "We are now entered into business," and turns the meeting over to the nurse. The secretary calls the roll. Those present, as they answer the roll call, tell how many births they have attended since the last meeting. Opportunity is given for the discussion of problems arising with recent deliveries and much can be learned from these discussions which often give the nurse a chance to do some of her best teaching. But each midwife would like to tell in detail about each birth she has attended, so the nurse has to keep a firm hand on the discussion to keep those recitals from taking up too much time.

At this point two questions almost invariably come up: "How can I make them notice me ahead of time?" and "How can I get my pay?" These questions are discussed and advice given. But the same questions come up over and over as if they were new. And over and over the midwives go when called, though they have had no previous notice and even though the patient may owe them for several previous deliveries.

At each meeting the nurse gives a simple demonstration for the midwives. It may be a demonstration of ways to make a baby breathe, how to make a bed pan of several thicknesses of newspapers, how to make and sterilize sanitary supplies of old clean rags which patients have on hand. After the nurse's demonstration the midwives practice the procedure with corrections and praise from the nurse. "One time the nurse said the way I did what she showed us was a better way than hers," Aunt Jeanie bragged, "and she had me teach it to the other grannies my way. I nearly burst wide open being proud."

Patience and care in teaching are essential, especially as some of the midwives cannot read. The nurse goes back to a brief review at subsequent meetings to make sure that what she taught is remembered and understood. Teaching must be done in terms of what the granny-midwives have to work with. For instance, in teaching how to sterilize equipment in covered pans in their ovens, the nurse explains that they can put into the oven at the same time a medium-sized potato. When the potato is baked, the articles to be sterilized are ready to be taken from the oven.

The midwives love to learn an occasional long medical term for something they have a simpler name for. But for the most part the nurse explains to them in simple terms and tries to make sure they understand any "big word" she gives them. Sometimes one of them will take pleasure in showing off her professional vocabulary. A doctor who was called by Granny Lou for a baby she delivered laughs about how she put him in his place with her use of medical terms. "I praised her for her carefulness," he said, "but in words I considered plain and simple. 'You were mighty smart,' I told her, 'to send for me when this baby started bleeding at the cord.' 'Maybe you calls it bleeding at the cord,' she replied. 'We calls it umbilical hemorrhage.' "

After the demonstration and practice comes the giving out of such supplies as are furnished by the State Department of Health. This replenishing of supplies is part of the bag inspection, or what the midwives call "the searching of the bag," to see if it measures up to required standards of cleanliness and contains the necessary articles of equipment, but contains nothing else. The nurse stresses a high standard of cleanliness and adequacy of supplies because of their importance to mothers and babies. Each article which is supposed to be in the bag is definitely needed and the lack of it may mean a case of "childbed fever" for the mother with perhaps resulting death. The lack of eye drops may mean blindness for the baby.

There is need to watch the bag for articles not supposed to be there, because such things may contaminate sterilized supplies. Nurses also watch for contraband in the midwife bag, because the grannies used to carry very little or nothing in the way of supplies except patent medicines, pills, brew of roots, herbs, etc.; homemade salves, all sorts of "remedies" with which they dosed their patients. They are now forbidden to do this. Nurses have learned to look under the removable lining of the bag. There may be found such things as coins tied into the corners of a handkerchief, a piece of rope, a box of snuff, a bottle of homemade tonic or "bitters," a rabbit's foot, or some other good luck charm.

During the "searching of the bag" at one such midwife meeting Aunt Roxy dramatized the inspection of her bag and enumerated its contents for the benefit of a visitor present.

"Now, nurse, honey, wait a minute till I spread out this paper to lay my things on." Aunt Roxy began.

"Now watch how tight shut my bag is to keep out the dust and germs. I open the outside and there are my things still shut up tight and clean in my lining to my bag. Look how white and clean the lining is. You got your little record book, nurse, honey, to check off my things as I name them? Here all the things rest in the pockets of the lining. My birth blanks and my pencil, my book of midwife orders from the Board, my book on how to tend mothers and babies, my midwife license. Pass that to the visiting lady so she can see how the Board writes down fresh every year that I got a right to be a granny-midwife. Don't that look proper legal and all?"

"That's fine, Aunt Roxy," interrupted the nurse, "but let's go right on with the inspection."

"Yes'm, begging your pardon. This bundle is my equipment case. On this side I keep the things I use my ownself personal. Wrapped up together here are my cap and gown and mask like folks wears in hospitals to do operations. After I use them, they get boiled and did up fresh and clean for the next time. Let me put them on, nurse, honey, to show our guest." With the nurse's nod of approval, "I first put on my cap and see that all of my hair is covered; then I put on my mask and see that all my mouth and nose is covered; then I scrub my hands and get ready for my gown. The gown is put in the bag folded wrong side outwards to keep it safer for the mother and the baby that's a-borning. I tie on my gown my ownself because my hands are clean and I don't want no dirty hands touching me. I used to think all these newfangled ideas about having to scrub my hands with a brush and wear all these things was foolishness, but I like it now. It makes my practice cleaner and safer. And then I do like to dress up suitable to any occasion.

"When I went through the motions of scrubbing, you saw my towel and the little bag with my soap, and brush, and nail picker. Now these other things belong to be used for the mother and the baby. There's lysol and that's boric acid powder, and cotton, and bandage cloth. Them's blunt scissors—no sharp points to stick the baby. There's the eye drops for the baby's eyes. These little packages done up separate has in each one a cord tie and a cord dressing like we make, and then sterilize out the germs. I used to tie the cord with any old string I could find, and mix grease and soot to put on it, and cover it with whatever rag was handy. It makes me tremble now to think how many germs I used. And I used to borrow the woman's scissors and wipe them on my apron and keep them under her mattress for nine days and—"

The nurse broke in with, "That's all very interesting, Aunt Roxy, but look at all the rest of these bags I have to inspect. Let's lift out the lining of your bag to show the visitor how it opens out flat to make a clean surface to put things on. Then you will be through." Out came the lining of the bag, and for a moment both the nurse and Aunt Roxy were speechless.

Then Aunt Roxy grabbed the nurse's hand that was reaching into the bag and shouted, "Don't touch that thing, honey! It's loaded, and you don't know the first thing about guns! That's Hebrew's pistol I been toting with me of late because I'm scared when I get called out in the middle of the night. I forgot to take it out my midwife bag this morning. Don't you worry, nurse, honey, I'll take it out now and tote it home separate in this stout paper sack. Will you-all excuse me out of the room a minute till I get the shame off me a little?"

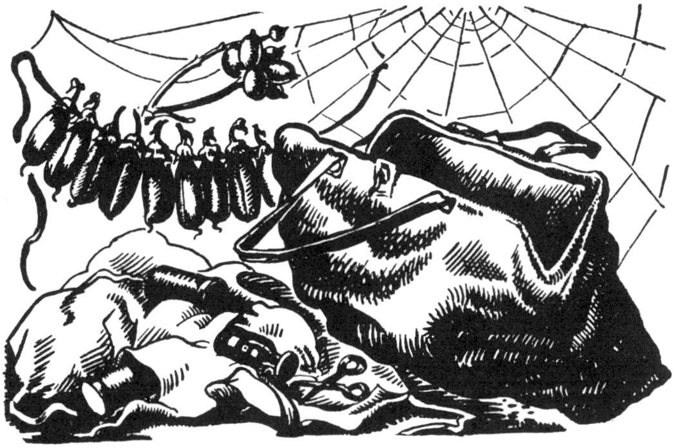

The Old Law and the New Law

"I TOLD her that's the New Law." Any nurse who works with midwives knows what that means, for she hears a lot about the Old Law and the New Law. To a Georgia midwife the New Law refers to any regulation by the Department of Health since the instruction and licensing of midwives in the State first began in 1925. The Old Law refers to midwife practices and beliefs which belong to the period before that and which still come in conflict with better practices which the midwife has been taught under the New Law.

Not only does the midwife have to learn procedures of sanitary and safe maternity care, but, if she is to have the coöperation of her patients, they also need to be educated in the ways of the New Law. The maternal and child health clinics are excellent opportunities for the public health nurses to teach the midwives and their patients together. Nurses encourage the midwives to come to these clinics. The midwife can be really helpful in the work of the clinic—a kind of nurse's aide. At the same time she can learn from the doctor and the nurses with her patients. The nurse with a heavy load of generalized public health work depends a great deal on her granny-midwives to tell her of expectant mothers and to help persuade them to come to the clinics. Sometimes the granny enlists the nurse's persuasive powers also, as in this case of a mother who saw no need for clinic attendance.

"I shore want you to see her," the midwife said. "She says she can't see no use going to the clinic or the doctor, 'cause her ma done had six babies and they ain't no doctor seen her yet. I told her the rules had changed under the New Law and I couldn't tend her if she didn't go to the doctor or the clinic and take a specification of urinate for a water tester and get a blood test to see if her blood was moral or did she have to take shots for herself and the baby so it will get born healthy."

A blood test for expectant mothers is required by Georgia law and whether or not the mother has had the blood test is to be indicated on the birth certificate. The nurses try to impress upon the midwives that the blood test is for the good of the mother so she can have treatment and safeguard her baby's health too; also, it indicates the need for the midwife to protect herself from infection when attending the mother. Grannies are not supposed to deliver a woman who does not have a paper certifying that she has had the required blood test from a private physician or at one of the venereal clinics held regularly in all Georgia counties. Some midwives are inclined to be negligent about this. Others are quite strict. One evening a county nurse heard an old car rattle up to the door of her home. A man came rushing in saying he had to have a blood test for his wife in a hurry. His wife was in labor and they had called the midwife. When she said she would not attend his wife unless she had her "strip," he bundled his wife into the car and came in a great hurry to get the matter fixed up.

One of the die-hards under the New Law is the old superstitions on the part of midwives and patients. The nurses do not pretend they succeed in eliminating all these ancient superstitious beliefs and practices. Nor do the midwives pretend that they have given up *all* their pet superstitions. The nurses tackle first and hardest those that are really harmful. For instance, it makes little difference, really, if the mother wears in childbirth the hat of her baby's father, or if there is an ax under her bed to ease the pain. But it makes a lot of difference if the midwife gives her tea made of dirt dauber's nests to make the pains stronger and hasten delivery. It is a serious matter too if she is kept on a starvation diet because she and her family, or the midwife, or the whole lot of them have a superstitious fear that anything but bread and coffee will make her ill. Or if they tie a black string around her waist to stop hemorrhage instead of sending for a doctor.

Sometimes there is a chance to discuss these superstitions with a group of midwives and their patients. On one such occasion a nurse was teaching midwives and prenatal clinic patients to make sterile pads of twelve thicknesses of large double sheets of newspaper spread flat and covered "slick and smooth" with old white rags which had been boiled clean. The paper and cloth were sewed and then sterilized at home in covered pans in a slow oven till a potato put in at the same time was done. One of the midwives said as they worked, "Under the Old Law we never done nothing like this. We just used any old things, dirty or clean. One time a woman told me to get a piece of old quilt off the porch. Old dog Tige was lying on it, but I kicked him off and put that dirty piece of quilt on the woman's bed. Scares me now to think what I done."

Then various old superstitions came up as part of the conversation. As these old beliefs wove in and out of the talk of the midwives and their patients, the nurse made them the basis of an excellent bit of teaching. "She didn't get preachy, neither," commented Aunt Tenny. "It was just a bunch of colored women with their nurse, talking about what was good things to do and what wasn't. I made me a list of what things they brought into their talk." Here is what she had on her list:

For the Mother:

Hemorrhage

Tie black string around the waist
Use cobwebs to coagulate the blood
Repeat—Ezekiel 16:3
16:6

Retained Placenta

Patient blow in a blue bottle
Set patient over hot chicken feathers

To ease body trouble—Sourwood root
Wild cherry bark tea

To make childbirth easier—Dogwood berries eaten raw

To guard against miscarriage—Tea of black haw roots

To bring on a miscarriage—Tansy tea

Somebody brought up the proper ritual for taking off the baby's cord. It should be done on the seventh day after birth. The cord must not be dropped on the floor and must be thrown straight into the middle of the fire, for if it touches the floor or the back of the fireplace the baby will have backache all its life. That was only a preface to mention of these other superstitious notions about baby care:

Teething—Rattle box plant pods on string around neck.
Narrow band of black velvet around the neck
Mole's foot around neck
Hog or dog tooth hung around neck
Briar root to chew on

Thrush—Persimmon bark tea
Rub baby's mouth with 9 leaves of sage
Let horse blow in baby's mouth

Birthmark removed by touching with dead man's hand.
Dried turtle heart tea for long life
Daddy-long-legs rolled in dough for chills
Hives—expose to sun three successive mornings
Colic—bone out of hog's foot
Grease knees with dish water to make baby walk early
Sugarberries (hackberries) dried and given to children as tidbits to do them good.

At another time a midwife club was discussing directions given to patients in preparation for home delivery. One midwife said she told the family to clear all the "junky stuff" out of the room. Another added that she told people to clean out the fireplace in the room where the baby would be born because they shouldn't take out the ashes in the mother's room nor carry fire from the room for six weeks after the baby's birth. To do either would make the mother sick.

Some superstitions which came up provoked argument among the midwives. Somebody said a baby born with a veil could foresee the future and see spirits. She said when little children stop, shiver, and "scrunch up" they are seeing spirits. One midwife said if the veil were taken off backward the child would not see boogers. Another argued that to dry the veil and make tea was a better way to cure him of seeing spirits. That provoked someone else to say that seeing spirits wouldn't hurt him none. Then a midwife who had delivered a baby with a veil ended the discussion by saying that she frequently asked the mother about this child born with a veil and the mother always told her it was no different from her other children.

Aunt Mary insisted that if a pregnant woman cleaned out a spring it would go dry. A man would have to clean it out after that before it would flow again, but he would have to wait till after the birth of the baby. Aunt Mary knew this was true because her sister did it to her spring. She would not let her sister draw water from her well for fear it too would go dry.

After this session on superstitions practiced freely under the Old Law, the midwives offered a surprise for the nurse, a song they had made up for their midwife club. To the lively tune of "Old Time Religion" they pledged themselves to follow the standards of the New Law.

Song of the Midwives
(Tune: *Old Time Religion*)

Chorus

(Sing first and use as chorus)

Give me that good old midwife meeting,
Give me that good old midwife meeting,
Give me that good old midwife meeting,
It is good enough for me.

We will wear our caps and gowns,
We will wear our caps and gowns,
We will wear our caps and gowns,
They are good enough for me.

Chorus

We'll use our soap and brushes,
We'll use our soap and brushes,
We'll use our soap and brushes,
They are good enough for me.

Chorus

We will always clean our nails,
We will always clean our nails,
We will always clean our nails,
It is good enough for me.

Chorus

We will always have a good bag,
We will always have a good bag,
We will always have a good bag,
It is good enough for me.

Chorus

Then we'll save our mothers and babies,
Then we'll save our mothers and babies,
Then we'll save our mothers and babies,
And it's good enough for me.

Chorus

Repeat chorus very softly

At another midwife club an even lengthier song composed by the midwives was presented as evidence that they practiced the teachings of the New Law.

Song of the Midwives

(Tune *As We Go Marching On*)

We aim to be good midwives of the State
We try hard to be up to date
To be on time to meetings and never to be late
As we go marching on.

Chorus

Glory, glory, hallehujah
Glory, glory, hallehujah
Glory, glory, hallehujah
As we go marching on.

We tell our mothers they should breathe fresh air
We show them what they need to prepare
We teach them what the baby should wear
As we go marching on.

We tell them plenty of water to drink,
About good food we cause them to think,
We say when tired, take of sleep a wink,
As we go marching on.

We put on water in a great big pot,
We know of this we must have a lot,
We boil it all, use some cool, some hot,
As we go marching on.

We put drops in the baby's eyes
Whether the mother laughs or cries,
The State for us the eye drops buys,
As we go marching on.

We report births and deaths and all
When anything is wrong, we the doctor call,
We hope we never from grace may fall,
As we go marching on.

We wear clean dress, clean cap, clean gown,
We have clean homes, clean yards, clean town,
We'll make our county of good renown,
As we go marching on.

Our county midwives are the best in the State,
They try hard to be up to date,
Are on time to meetings and never are late,
As we go marching on.

After they had sung their new song for her and gone on their way, the nurse said, "You know, under the circumstances in which they often work I could not do as well as they do. No, I don't fool myself into thinking that the old superstitions are all but extinct in actual practice. Last week I was called to see two babies who had a terrible rash. I found their families had been giving them hot tea made from moldy corn fodder. A neighbor had said it was just good for babies in a general way. The attendant midwife hadn't thought it could do any harm. An intelligent, educated woman fed her little girl a fried mouse to cure her from 'branching in the bed,' as our midwives call it. How much of the Old Law is mingled with the New Law in practice of midwifery by the grannies? Only direct supervision of each delivery would tell. And the public health nurse in Georgia carries too heavy a load for that. She does make home visits to expectant and new mothers. She does what teaching she can in the home and at clinics, hoping the mother will come to expect and insist upon the best care the midwife can give. She gives the midwife what supervision and help she can."

And what does the midwife do for the nurse? For one thing she gives help in other services than maternal health. A nurse who is trying to educate people to early diagnosis and treatment of tuberculosis welcomes this note from one of her midwives:

> My sister's little boy has been exposed to T.B. So will you kindly do me a favor the next time you all have

clinic there. Write him a card and x-ray his chest. Please give him the patch test. Your considerations appreciated.

Where progress in venereal disease education seems slow such a message from a midwife as this is indeed a help in finding cases who need to go to Augusta or Savannah to rapid treatment centers or for slower treatment at their own clinics.

> For the comenity (community) sick (sake) will you all send........ to Ag (Augusta) Georgia for her to get well of her disenses (diseases) don't she Spoil this country for she officle bad threw here.

Another midwife note says a patient has just come back from the "Horse-pillow," and thus saves the nurse a long trip into the country.

Nurses say they learn from the midwives—largely things of the spirit. One nurse said she had learned from them to have what they call "long patience," a necessary quality for one in a public health program where much is a slow matter of education. Another said she had learned that people of different races and social levels could mutually respect and like one another. Still another said she had learned that intelligence is not a matter of education, that a person of superior knowledge can learn from one who has had experience, that she had learned to look at both sides of questions that come up.

Miss Laura Blackburn, who has had long experience with granny-midwives, summarizes in her "What the

Midwife Has Taught the Nurse"[1] some of the things nurses have told her they learned from the granny-midwives by working with them.

"I have learned," said one nurse, "the simplicity of dignity and the dignity of simplicity." "I have watched the midwives," said another, "and have come to realize the value of justice tempered with mercy, and the power of group thinking." One nurse said, "I have developed poise by watching them, have learned to talk in public by getting experience with them, and their ready response has taught me that the listener has as much to do with the success of a speech as does the speaker." A practically minded young nurse said, "I have learned how to meet difficult and unexpected situations with equanimity and to use what can be found around a house instead of being either helpless or demanding that the family buy things which they are not able to afford."

"A nurse who was doing a good piece of teaching said, "I have learned from the midwives how important it is to have graphic and picturesque speech in teaching and that demonstrations and dramatizations can not be overestimated." Others have said, "We have learned lessons of tolerance, kindness, generosity of giving and sharing, sympathy and understanding." Others that faith is necessary, beautiful, powerful, highly desirable and practical. Contentment with very little is a wonderful thing. A mature nurse said, "I think the most outstanding thing I have learned from the midwives is their attitude toward sex. . . . They are so kind in their attitude and treatment of these poor little unmarried prenatals. They are so gentle and understanding; they don't see anything so wrong about it—just unfortunate."

[1] Blackburn, Laura, "What the Midwife Has Taught the Nurse," *Public Health Nursing.*

Even those nurses who are at first intolerant of the midwives when they start to work with them seldom fail to fall under the spell of their simple charm. One such nurse laughingly said, "My midwives have conjured me out of my intolerance. Now I find myself stanchly defending them against undue criticism, explaining them to doctors, to civic clubs, to any who don't give them what I consider their dues. Only witchcraft could have worked that change in me. Call it whatever you like. I am proud of any least improvement my midwives make."

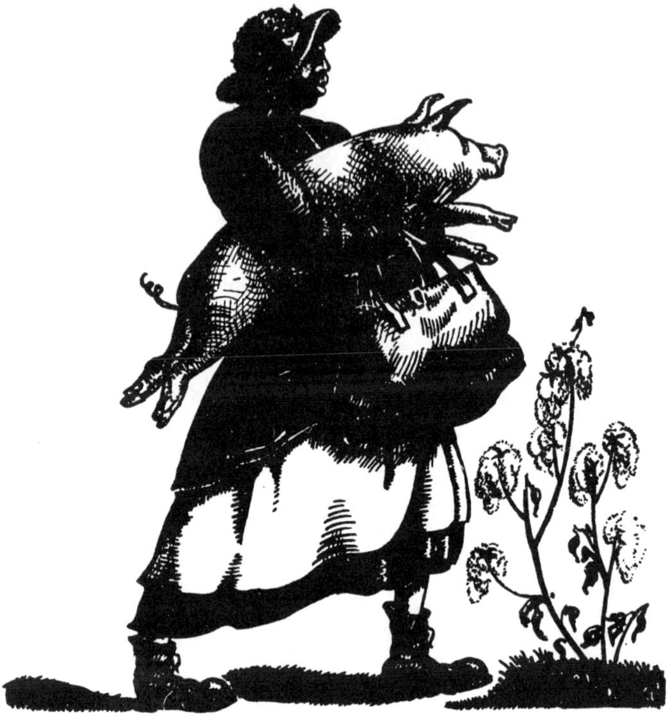

Two Questions at the Last

"TWO QUESTIONS I save to the last." A midwife was explaining how she organized her work at a home delivery. "After the baby gets born and I got the mother and it tended to good, and all the other things done I'm supposed to do, then just before I start to leave I ask them two questions at the last: 'What you name the baby?' and 'What about my pay?' "

This question of "what about my pay?" is an ever recurring one for the midwife, and all too often there is no satisfactory answer for it—or maybe no answer at all. It has been thus through the years.

Countless times during the years when he was Director of the Division of Maternal and Child Health of the Georgia Health Department the midwives asked Dr. Joe P. Bowdoin, "How can I get my pay?" It was under his direction that the instruction and supervision of midwives in Georgia was begun. He was devoted to his midwives and would brook no undue criticism of them.

He was their last court of appeal and they wrote him hopefully about their troubles. One of the most frequent subjects of this midwife correspondence of his was the matter of pay for delivering babies. One of Dr. Joe's favorite stories from the files of these letters concerns the midwife who was given a pig in payment for her services. She carried the pig home with her and put it into a pen. But in the night the pig broke out of the pen and returned to its former place of abode. The man then refused to give it back to the midwife, because, he said, he had discharged his obligations when he gave her the pig the first time. The midwife wrote to Dr. Joe, asking him to set the matter straight for her.

There are innumerable stories of things the midwives receive instead of cash payment. One old granny said that all she ever got for one case was a large pink conch shell. It was pretty, but it is bad luck to own a conch shell. So she left it in the graveyard for an ornament as she passed through.

Another was given a big china platter with a rabbit painted on it. "A nice dish," she said, "but it fairly turned my stomach to eat off a platter that had a rabbit on it big as life and with the fur on."

Someone took a bushel of meal in payment, only to find when she got home that the meal was full of weevils and fit for nothing but chicken feed.

A man offered to do plowing to settle his debt to the midwife and she accepted. Then she found that he had no mule or other work animal to do plowing with. A woman who could not sew suggested sewing for the midwife to pay for the baby.

"The best pay I ever got for my granny work," said Aunt Kansas, "was a speckled bird dog pup. It never looked like much when it was given to me, but I took it on account of it was that or nothing for pay. Then it turned out to be a fine bird dog that took prizes and that bird hunters from the big cities would pay good money to hunt with. It had fine pups, too, that we could sell for twenty-five dollars a piece after my youngest boy trained them. In the years before she was killed with a truck backing over her, old Babe had nineteen pups. We figured one time that she brought in, all told, around six hundred dollars. The best pay I ever got for catching any baby."

Aunt Charity says one person paid her with a pair of geese, another with a few hens, still another with a barrel of onions collected by her relatives as surplus commodities on relief. Somebody else said to Aunt Charity, "I'll pay you when I thrash my cats"—meaning never.

Some families pay the midwife just nothing at all, some half the fee, and some all of it. There are families who pay for the last baby when another is coming and they again need the service of the midwife. Some owe for children born years ago. Aunt Vina said, "If I could collect what's owing me, I wouldn't need any old age pension. It ain't the ones that owes me that's paying the pension neither. They ain't the kind that pays taxes."

The amount of the fee charged by midwives and their success in collecting vary with communities as well as with individuals. They say that people are better about paying them now than when they charged only two dollars for a delivery. They say also that they are paid better since midwives are licensed. "Ain't no two ways about it," they declare. "We gets our pay more and oftener since we been on the Board. Lots of folks figure they have to pay, because they think the Health Department is behind us grannies."

People are more likely to think this in counties that have a county nurse, who holds prenatal clinics. At these clinics patients who wish to use a midwife for delivery are given a slip of paper stating that the prospective mother has had a blood test, a thorough examination, and has permission to call a midwife. On this "strip," as the midwives call it, ten dollars is suggested as the fee for the granny-midwife. The grannies say that helps them to get their money. Nurses encourage people to pay for delivery of their babies and urge the grannies to be more hard-boiled about getting their money.

But for all their grumbling about not getting paid, they will keep on going on cases without pay. The midwife may say, "I done caught six babies for that trifling set and they ain't paid me for nary one yet." But when the next call comes from that same family with the promise, "I shore pay you cotton picking time," she goes, "for a woman in her misery done sent for me."

Traditionally, the midwife's service may be had for very little, almost for the asking. Certainly no midwife ever entered her profession for the money there is in it.

Sometimes the midwife has occasion to grumble about the response to her question "What you name the baby?" Some families are too slow choosing a name. The midwife is required by law to file a birth certificate with the local registrar within ten days after the birth. "Us grannies got to turn in our birth mints," they complain. "So we need for folks to hurry up and name the baby. Did you ask does they ever let us do the naming? Maybe once in a coon's age. But just any kinfolks or neighbors that didn't lift a finger to do nothing for the baby, they get to pick out the name."

The granny-midwives and their nurses tell many stories about people naming their babies. Among their favorites are the stories of why a girl baby was named Vacate, why another was called Angel Blue, or an especially charming baby was given the name Precious Character.

One man who wanted a son kept naming his girls Willie for himself until there were in his family Willie Jane, Willie Sue, Willie Mae, Willie Kate, and Willie Bertha. When a boy finally arrived, the father proposed to name him William. But the mother refused. "I got enough Willies," she said. "This baby's name is Bishop Moore."

A mother who liked the name Kate gave all her daughters the middle name of Kate. There were Rosie Kate, Tommy Kate, Jessie Kate, Missouri Kate.

To anyone who is incredulous about midwives' and nurses' stories of babies named Annie Cute or Strawberry Smith a look into the birth records for both white and colored babies will be proof that the naming stories are not fictional at all. Results of today's unprecedented interest in other countries and cities are found in names taken from records filed with the State Department of Health. A few such names are:

French Works	Emma Line Ireland
Warm London	India Printup
Roosevelt National	United States Campbell
England M. Ready	Travel Dennark

There are other unique names which derive from items of food and drink. Among these some stir memories of preration days:

Georgia Bacon	Tea Gowan
Florida Sweets	Sugar Blanks

Strawberry Smith	Fed Wright
Coca Cola Gamble Baggett	China Rice
Virginia Ham	

When the midwife finally gets the baby's name, that is only part of her troubles ended. The birth certificates —"birth mints" some midwives call them—can cause a heap of trouble. Those grannies who cannot write have some one else fill out the required blanks while they touch the pen. Any who can write at all insist, as a matter of pride, on filling out their own "birth mints." Things go very well for those who write easily. For those who can barely write it is indeed a struggle. Nurses furnish sample blanks and give lessons and practice on filling out birth certificates correctly. Still the local registrars have their share of grief over scarcely legible and barely intelligible records. One nurse jokingly said that a registrar of vital statistics thought any midwife was a good one if she turned in promptly records which he could read and interpret.

Some of the registrars have what the midwives call "short patience" with their phonetic spelling and their labored attempts to write. One old granny says her registrar often gets fractious and talks rough to her about the "birth mints" she gives him. She says, "When I go to take him my birth mints, I stop outside the door and I look to the Lord and say, 'Do Jesus, don't let him get so fractious today and fuss at me so bad.' And maybe he talks nice that day. Then I stop when I come out the door and I say, 'Thank you, Jesus. He wasn't so bad today.' "

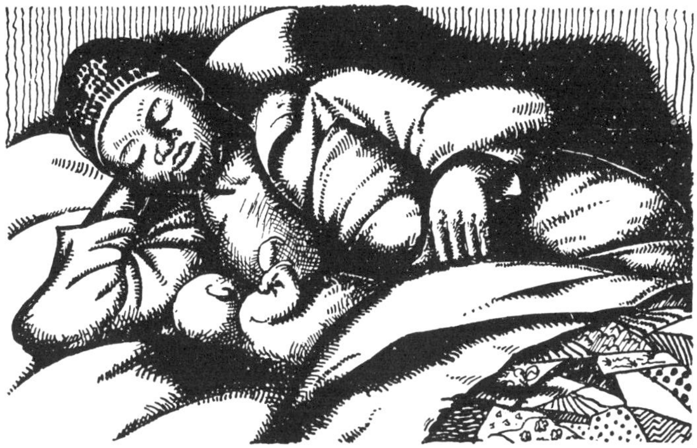

Come and Bring the Warmer

"YES'M, I waited here all the forenoon, but that seemed like the quickest way to get this message to you in person." The farmer who had been waiting at her office several hours while the public health nurse was working at school clinics in the country handed her a folded scrap of rough tablet paper on which had been printed in pencil I GOT A PRE-BORN BABY. COME AND BRING THE WARMER. Attempts to spell *incubator* had been scratched out.

"From one of my midwives, Granny Lou," the nurse explained, "and she wants the incubator that the State Department of Health placed here at the health center for the use of premature babies."

"Yes'm, I know," the farmer answered. "This baby

belongs to a colored family on my place. A good family too and been with us for years. We'd like it mighty well if you could save this baby, for their oldest, their only other boy, got killed in the army. Our youngest did too. Seems like that makes my wife and me more foolish about babies, white or colored. My wife said tell you she would help Margaret—this baby's mother—and the grandmother manage the baby in the incubator. Seems like she and Margaret can't do enough for each other since they lost their boys in common. She's down there now with Granny Lou to help keep folks from handling or bothering the baby till you get there."

As the nurse checked the incubator to see that it was in order, he went across the square to do a few errands at the stores. When all was ready, he carried the incubator downstairs to the nurse's car, commenting on its pretty pink color. The nurse told him that some people objected to the incubators painted white, because they were reminded of coffins. So the nurses painted the incubators various pastel colors and stenciled on nursery pictures of rabbits, ducks, etc., to give them a more cheerful appearance.

"No matter what color to me," was the response, "so long as it keeps a baby alive for a woman with a boy killed in the war. Now you go ahead and I'll trail you in my car so's to be there to help you if you get stuck on these muddy country roads." And the "warmer" was on its way to Margaret's "pre-born" baby.

One of the great needs for these incubators furnished by the public health service is in the care of premature multiple births. A public health nurse in a recent issue of *Georgia's Health* tells this story of triplets in whose survival she had a personal part:

> Lenora, Elnora and Honora are my pride and joy. No one thought they would live. Helping keep them alive was a challenge to put any nurse on her mettle. Johnny, the mother, is a young Negro woman who lives with her elderly parents. When "the baby" took so long coming, Johnny was taken to the hospital. The family was aghast at the appearance of three little brown mites when only one was expected. They refused to believe they would live. The physician patiently explained to Pecoalia, the grandmother, how to care for Johnny and the three tiny girls but she seemed too dazed to understand instructions. When the children were ready to go home, I arranged to take them in the Health Department incubator to avoid exposing them and to leave the incubator in the home.
>
> I did not give the family many instructions on care of the babies that first morning because they had to get used to the fact that the babes were alive and at home. I did show them how to mix the formula, how to feed them and keep them warm. I warned them against letting people open the incubator. People were kind and interested in the struggle to keep Lenora, Elnora and Honora alive. They furnished supplies, food and help. The mechanic at the county shop made a stove similar to a Sterno stove, using a Tetley's tea can for the alcohol, to heat the formula. A milk company furnished a year's supply of milk. The family's original consternation at the appearance of the three gave way to great pride and Pecoalia and Johnny devoted themselves wholeheartedly to the care of the babies. The Regional nurse and the Health Department physician helped me keep the babies under constant supervision.
>
> One stifling summer day, I arrived to find the babies

in a baby bed instead of the incubator and the room unbearably hot. Pecoalia and Johnny decided the incubator looked "too much like a coffin" and had decided to build a fire and keep the whole room at the proper incubator temperature. Besides, the grandmother said, "It helps keep folks from visitin' 'em." How they stood that room so hot during July, August and September is a mystery to me. But the babies are thriving. They weighed around 3 pounds each at birth and now average approximately 6 pounds apiece. The triplets were in fair condition at birth and they owe their lives, I think, to that factor mixed with the coöperation of family and interested persons and a great deal of prayer.

Sometimes it is difficult to find anyone to give home care to the premature baby, especially where there is a woman power shortage as there was in one particular farm home where the youngest member of the family was a two-day-old boy weighing four and one-half pounds. His two and one-half-pound sister had lived only a day. Though heat was essential to his life, the weather was bitter cold. He and his mother occupied one of the three beds in a large, drafty, combination sitting room-bedroom, heated only by a small wood stove. The unceiled little farmhouse was not built for cold weather.

The mother was weak and worn from the ordeal of giving birth to premature twins. The rest of the family was totally masculine—three boys aged three, nine, and fourteen, and the father, who was sick with fatigue and dazed from two days and nights without sleep. The only close neighbor woman was good and kind, but also deaf and dumb, with a small grandchild to care for. The mother had always done everything for her family of men, and they were bewildered and helpless without her.

The nurse scoured the country but could not find a woman to stay with the family or a female relative who could or would come. All the while the mother steadfastly refused to allow the baby to be put into an incubator.

A message to the State Health Department brought a public health doctor and an incubator. Together he and the nurse visited the home and found the male members of the family huddled around the stove. The mother had the baby in bed with her close to her side under the covers. She protested pathetically that she could "do for the baby" by propping herself up on her elbow and could keep him warm with her body. But the doctor persuaded her finally to let them put the baby in the incubator where he would be protected from infection and cold.

The doctor prescribed a feeding schedule, and then came the question of teaching someone to care for the baby until the mother was strong enough to be taught herself. The father was obviously the only choice, though he was frightened of the responsibility and declared that he knew nothing about babies. In spite of his distaste for such apparel, the nurse tied one of her clean white aprons on him and the two of them tackled the mysteries of premature infant care. He watched every step carefully from the initial hand scrubbing to putting those drops of milk *on top* of the baby's tongue with a medicine dropper. Though he was frightened because the baby was so little, he caught on quickly. The mother was worried because she said, "He ain't never so much as didied one of our younguns." But he did well indeed. His big hands were rough and scarred, but he handled his son as gently as a woman. At the mother's request he pushed the incubator up against the side of her bed where she could watch the baby through the glass. Each time after that, when the nurse stopped in to see that all was going well with the baby, the father beamed with pride that he could "do for his family" in the woman power shortage.

Other premature babies are often well blessed with attentive relatives and neighbors. In fact, an incubator baby may become something of a local exhibit. Not long ago a private physician called the health center in his county, saying he had delivered premature triplets to a colored mother in the country. One of the babies had died at birth, but the remaining two needed incubator care.

The nurse taught the grandmother how to manage the incubator and care for the babies. When she returned the next day to check on the success of feeding directions, neighbors—white and colored—were streaming in and out of the house to look at the babies in the incubator. On her second return trip the company was still coming and going. As she opened the incubator to care for the baby, she had to move a little cardboard box with a hole in the top of it and a sign which said,

GIVE TO THE TRIBUTES IN THE NAME OF JESUS. The box rattled when picked up, so evidently there had been contributions.

Not only does the public health nurse give instructions and help in home care of premature infants but also it is part of her duty to teach her midwives to recognize when a baby is premature or has some other condition that indicates incubator care. She tries to teach the midwives how important it is to notify her at once when they deliver such a baby, so there will be as little delay as possible in starting the kind of attention it needs if it is to live.

At a midwife meeting for such instructions the midwives discussed what was done in the way of premature care before incubators were available for home use. "Mostly they didn't know to treat them no different to other babies," one midwife said. "And they just lived or died according as they were able. Mostly the granny-midwives and the family the baby belonged to were ignorant of what needed to be done, and they wouldn't have had the right things to work with nohow."

Molly Baker indignantly rose to the defense of her mother, who had been a midwife. "My mama, Aunt Molly folks called her, was more knowing and clever than most, I reckon; but she didn't give up trying on account of what she had or didn't have to work with. Did you see the Judge go past here a while back? Well, he was a little bitty weak thing born two months ahead of time. Wizzled up and weighing not four pounds when my mama caught him.

"He was such a sorry looking excuse for a baby that his daddy and his granddaddy both said, 'Might as well lay him in his box and give up. It can't live and no use to fool yourself thinking he can. It's same as gone already.'

"My mama said, 'You hush your mouths, and get back to your own part of the house from under my feet. I aim to save this baby for Mis' Beatrice or die trying.' And she took and wrapped the little bitty thing in soft flannel cloths next to his skin with wool blankets wrapped around him outside of the flannel. Then she found an old close-woven picnic basket with a lid and made a warm nest of bedclothes in it and laid the baby in with fruit jars of warm water all around—kept warm all the time. She wouldn't let nobody touch him but herself, and she fed him mother's milk with an eye dropper. For weeks she stood over him until he was the right age to be born and had picked up enough weight to be treated like a natural baby. They lived out on the plantation where the Judge lives now, and we lived where I do now on their place. Only where I live was Mama's when she died, and she left it to me. Mama always felt like the Judge was partly hers because she helped him live. And he turned out to be Mis' Beatrice's only child she ever had.

"When the Judge fell heir to his daddy's property he deeded over to Mama in her name the house she lived in with four acres of ground and give it to her for a present. That was fine with Mama till she found out the taxes came in her name too. Then she raised objections. When the house wasn't hers she lived in it free from rent or any cost. Now it belonged to her she had to pay taxes.

"The colored school teacher talked with her and said propertied citizens had to take more responsibilities like taxes and things. Mama said, 'That high-minded talk sounds good, but it don't make me want to pay no taxes.' So she made the Judge pay the taxes right on as long as she lived. He said that was little enough reward to her this side of heaven after what she done to keep him in this world.

"Mama has climbed that long road to heaven but I do hope she can lean over the edge and see this here baby warmer, for not many folks are clever as Aunt Molly was to save pre-born babies with just whatever things they can find about the place. How proud she would feel that all us granny midwives got to do now is send our supervisor and supreme a message to come and bring the warmer when we catch a pre-born baby."

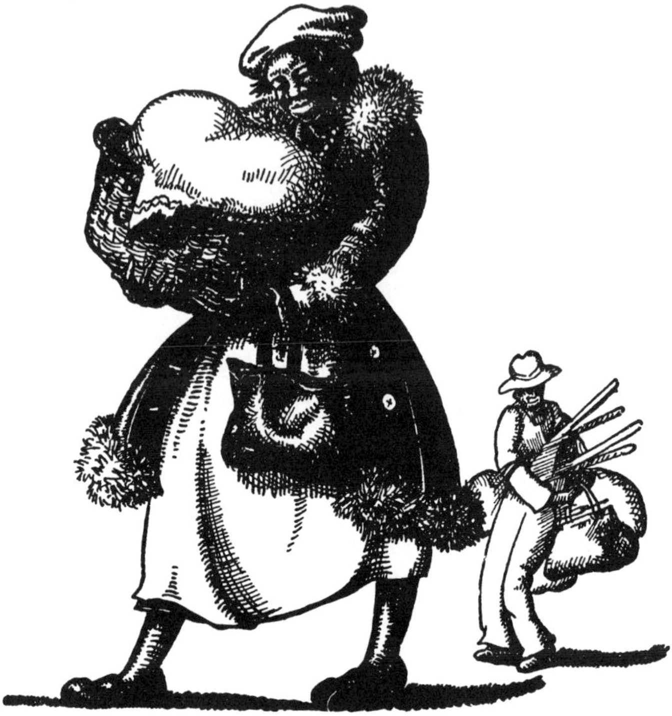

Picnic Lunch and Mary Belle's Picture

"No, I don't make a motion to approve the minutes the secretary just read. I rose up to say they ain't proper minutes of this Midwife Club," Aunt Molly Baker objected. "That last part just uses up a lot of words, and ain't got nothing to do with the business we transacted at our last meeting. Write that part off, and then they will be proper minutes to approve."

As Aunt Molly's remarks indicate, the approval of the minutes of a midwife club meeting is no perfunctory matter. All of the midwife clubs keep records of all their meetings, and the minutes of the previous time are read and approved at each meeting. The clubs are very proud of the records they keep and each page has to be considered suitably written before it is made a part of the record. The following is an example of a page from such a record, a copy of the minutes of a special meeting held by the Schley County Midwife Club:

Ellaville, Ga. Schley County
12/1/44

The Schley County mid wife Club.

We the Schley county mid wives meet 12/1/44 with our nurses of Griffin, Ga. Miss Vera Mingleduff, Mrs Anna Brown. Also two nurses from the State of Texas. An two nurses of Buenavista, Ga. Mrs. Heart an Mrs Merphia. Opening Song no. 49. Sub. Bless be the Tides that binds our hearst in Christan love. prair by Sister Vina Gay. Song no 35 don't let it be said too late. we all then enjoyed an old fashion basket dinner served as a picnic After witch entered in business. All reports was made Sister Clara Williams reported Two births. Sister Eliza Terry reported Three births. Sister Mary B. Smith reported one birth Sister Vera Swans repoted Not any. Sister Mattie Green reported Not any. A pitcure of a delivery was made by Sister Mary B. Smith The pitcure was good. The class then looked at an example made by Mrs. Vera Mingleduff which was very helpfull. We them sang no 103. Sub. when them Saints go Marching in. The ordance was dismissed by Sister Vina Gay. Sister Vina Gay pres, Sister Mattie Green Vice. pres. Sister Vera Swans. Sect. Sister Eliza Terry Tres.

The special occasion recorded here was in addition to the regular December meeting to be held later in the month. On this special day the Midwife Club had as their guests to an old-fashioned basket dinner, spread in picnic style, the Regional Supervisory Nurse and her assistant, two nurses who hold itinerant venereal clinics in their county, and two other guests listed in the minutes as nurses from the State of Texas. As I am neither a nurse nor from the State of Texas, I was a little surprised to be so designated in the record, which was otherwise factually accurate.

When the guests arrived at the health center on the outskirts of town at the appointed hour only one of the hostesses had come. That was to be expected, for their homes were scattered all over the county and they had to manage the best way they could for rides to the county seat town. We were quite impressed with the importance of the occasion when the midwife there to greet us told us that she had just come home especially for the occasion from New York City where she had been visiting her son recently discharged from the Army. During the same trip she had visited others of her children in Florida before going on to New York. She was full of interesting talk about the places where she had been, but was happy to be back at home with her family. She is the mother of nineteen children, sixteen of whom are living, the youngest nine-year-old twin girls. She has eleven grandchildren, three of whom are now living with her. Seven of her children are at home, one away at school, one in the Army, the others married and living in her own county, in New York, and in Florida. She said with her own children and her grandchildren she had a whole cowpen full of little girls at her house.

After a while other midwives began to drift in with their baskets and to ask one another if Aunt Vina was coming. Some thought not, as she had not been well. Two of the guests decided to go for Aunt Vina, since she lived there in the county seat. Aunt Vina is a retired midwife, nearly eighty years old, but she still attends the meetings of her Midwife Club. In fact, she is honorary president of the club. Her neighbors pointed the way to Aunt Vina's house hidden by shrubbery and trees. Aunt Vina was not ready to go. She said she had to primp a little more. But she gave us half a caramel cake her daughter had made for her. We picked up one of Aunt Vina's friends, who asked us to stop by for her friend, Mattie. Mattie had visitors from Alabama and couldn't come till later, though she sent her basket of lunch by us.

In due time Aunt Vina arrived carrying an empty basket with a carefully folded towel in the bottom of it. Friends took her basket and helped her off with her wraps. Then Aunt Vina with a dramatic flourish pinned on her bosom a resplendent purple and gold retired midwife badge. Of course guests who were not nurses or midwives asked about it, and Aunt Vina described the ceremony at the Midwife Club when she formally retired and this badge was given her. "Giving me what I earned," said Aunt Vina. "The Lord laid this burden of granny-midwife on me when I was thirty-two and I toted it many a year. Through the years I carried the burden as best I knowed, though my best weren't always good enough."

Aunt Vina interrupted her own midwifery talk to announce that she was taking up a collection to help put a top on her church and that all contributions would be welcome, since she had to have fifty dollars collected by the second Sunday in January. After the collection the midwives sat around talking with the nurses about people they knew, and health and maternity problems in the county. "We're waiting for Sister Mary Belle," one of them explained. "She's the chairman of arrangements for this occasion and naturally we can't go ahead till she gets here."

Finally Sister Mary Belle came bustling in with a heaped up basket, her husband following with another load which she bundled out of sight. The husband went on his way; and, with the chairman now present, affairs could officially go forward. The chairman chose two midwives to help her, while the older midwives and the guests looked on. The picnic lunch was spread on Mary Belle's white table cloth with a little Christmas tree set in the middle. One of the guests was allowed to carve Mary Belle's roast chicken, and the midwives teased the carver. They said she wouldn't make a good stepmother because she cut the slices of chicken so thin. Plenty of good food came out of the midwife baskets. Fried chicken, sweet potatoes, pumpkin pie, sweet potato pie, fried apple and peach pies ("puffs" Aunt Vina called them), stuffed eggs, biscuits, corn bread, loaf bread, all kinds of cake—and Mary Belle's famous sugar pudding!

The nurses made their contributions to the picnic too. A huge angel food cake, sandwiches, a big basket of fruit, thermos jugs of coffee. The midwives were pleased no end, but they protested, "Oh you didn't need to do this. You ought not gone to the trouble. We fixed plenty for everybody." Indeed they had.

With towels from the baskets over our knees for napkins we waited expectantly. But midwife meetings always begin with a devotional service, and picnics are no exception. Everybody sang "Blest Be the Tie," and then Aunt Vina offered her own version of the Lord's Prayer with such variations and additions as it pleased her to make. The next song, "Don't Let It Be Said 'Too Late,'" was announced as a duet by Mary Belle and her sister Vera. The others hummed accompaniment for the first stanza and then could not resist joining in full voice.

The guests were served first by virtue of being guests. Each hostess was eager to have her food tasted and complimented. Each did not, however, urge her own cooking on others, but courteously urged guests to eat what her sister midwives had brought. "You don't know what's good if you ain't tasted Mary Belle's sugar pudding." "Sister Clara sure can't carry her stack cake back home not touched." "Now you know it ain't a true picnic if you don't eat no stuffed eggs. Sister Vera does make the best ones."

There was much talk of favorite foods and how to cook certain things. Tales of other picnic occasions went the rounds. Mary Belle and Vera told how their mother used to take her food to basket dinners in a little old trunk. They laughingly described their efforts when children to get a taste of their mother's picnic food before they left home, because other people always ate up their mother's food so quickly at a picnic, leaving them to eat what was brought by poorer cooks. Aunt Clara told of going to an all-day singing with dinner on the grounds when the mosquitoes were so bad that to keep them off the children rolled in the pennyroyal growing near by. Grown people crushed the leaves and rubbed on their arms and faces. Aunt Vina, peeling an orange and eating it slowly segment by segment, remembered a Christmas seventy-two years before when she and five little brothers and sisters had one orange. Aunt Mattie remembered seeing a barrel of fancy piece candy in a store one Christmas when it seemed to her more candy than she knew was in the world. "Other things that you had are good as candy," reminded Aunt Clara, "boiled peanuts, sugar cane to chew, and watermelon. But I reckon candy looks better when you're little, don't it, though?"

In the clearing up after lunch, leftovers were exchanged freely to take home. The other midwives gave

Aunt Vina enough to fill her basket which she had expectantly brought empty. They carefully divided the fruit brought by one of the nurses, divided it according to the number each had at home to share it. They did up packages with slices of their cakes for their guests to carry home with them. Two midwives came after lunch was over. One of them had to do a washing before she could start. The other had been out on a case the night before.

With the clearing up all done, and the late arrivals fed, the meeting "entered into business." The number of births since the last meeting in November were reported. But that was only a preliminary. The real business of the midwives at this meeting was to impress upon their guests how much they needed and wanted a public health nurse in their county. For some years they had a county nurse and then the war deprived them of her. Because of the shortage of nurses available for public health service it had been impossible as yet to replace their nurse. They had repeatedly been told that, but they thought it would not do any hurt to try again, to try a little harder to impress especially their Regional Supervisor as to how much they had learned from their former nurse and how much they wanted and needed a successor for her. To demonstrate how much and how well they had learned what the nurse had taught them as midwives, Mary Belle "made a picture" of a home delivery with her sister midwives as a watchful and critical part of the audience. The rest of us were carried along with the drama of it.

Mary Belle had made a dramatic entrance when she arrived. A little late, the whole group waiting on her, she came rustling in with the freshest of white uniforms and cap in contrast to the other midwives' dark winter clothing. She carried a beautiful picnic basket, and was followed by her husband loaded down with a large doll, bed, bedding, midwife bag and other paraphernalia which were quickly put out of sight. Now after the picnic, Mary Belle brought out all these things to set the stage for her "picture" of a home delivery as she would manage it. Mary Belle played all the parts throughout except that dolls represented the mother and baby.

As the "picture" began, Mary Belle had been sent for, and arrived just after the patient's husband had gone to his work. The prospective mother was alone with her mother-in-law, and Mary Belle took charge at once.

By implication it soon became evident that the mother-in-law was worried about the birthing of this first grandchild of hers and did not completely trust Mary Belle. She would have preferred an older midwife and one who did not look and act so sprucy and up-to-date. Sensing this, Mary Belle was very reassuring and polite, and diplomatically kept the mother-in-law busy, but at errands which kept her out of the patient's room most of the time. The problem of dealing with the mother-in-law was further complicated by the fact that she was totally deaf "from being picked up in a cyclone and whirled around six times before she hit the earth again." All communication with her had to be written or relayed through the patient, whose lips she could read.

The girl had gone to bed with her clothing on, so Mary Belle got her into a nightgown and made the bed in exactly the prescribed fashion. She found under the pillow the money the husband had left for the midwife. Putting the money back carefully, she whispered an aside, "That's got to come out from under there before I go home."

That remark prompted comments from the sidelines. And from that time on through the course of Mary Belle's dramatization there were comments and questions from the other midwives. Mary Belle wove them into the drama of what she was doing and saying. They became the comments and questions of well-meaning but ignorant neighbors who dropped in during the course of the day and whom Mary Belle answered patiently and carefully and then tactfully got rid of. Such was Mary Belle's sense of drama and her ability to act that she made the whole thing dramatic and interesting even to the nurses who had taught her much of what she was doing. And Mary Belle left out nothing which she had been taught as correct procedure for a normal home delivery.

But she was not too perfect to be convincing. Once her patience and tact with the mother-in-law wore thin. Mary Belle was rubbing the newborn baby with oil, fussing playfully about it's being such a "little bitty thing to fool with." The mother-in-law demanded that she wash the baby with soap and water. Forgetting that the woman couldn't hear her, Mary Belle simply blurted out, "Don't be so picayunish. Instructions from the nurses under the New Law says to oil this baby now and wash him the next day. That's what I aim to do."

But for all her following out completely to the letter the instructions under the New Law, there crept into Mary Belle's "picture" some practices which belonged to the Old Law. When she was taking care of the baby, she explained carefully that the cord must be dressed up the baby's stomach. "To turn the water up so he won't make a branch in the bed every night." Also she went back to the Old Law for the "white cloth fried in cow tallow flavored with camphor and turpentine and laid on hot," which she prescribed if the patient should have abdominal cramps within the next few days.

The father arrived from his day's work just before Mary Belle went home. So she showed him his new son, and left him a headful of instructions to be carried out before she came again the next day. With her hand on the door knob, she turned back to say, "Notify me immediately if anything goes wrong, so I can see if she needs a doctor. If she gets infected everything is laid on my shoulders." Then a last word to the new mother, "Feeling all right, honey? Ain't got no bad headache? No stars thrashing before your eyes?"

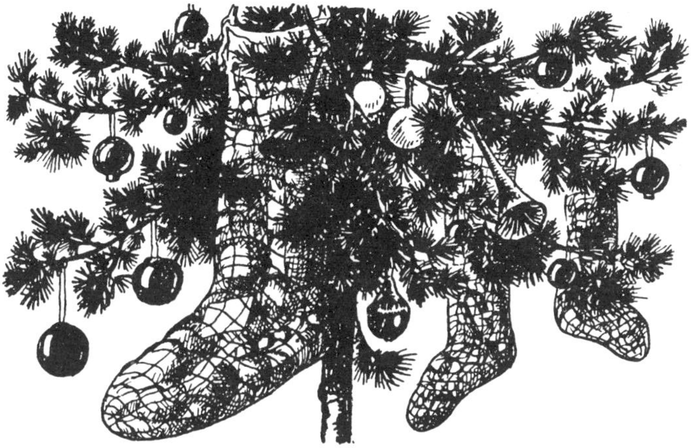

Christmas Party in the Courtroom

"IN MARCH the Butts County midwives were still talking about their Christmas party. As their little group gathered for the monthly meeting, they were seeing the big courtroom of the county courthouse not in its actual empty bareness but dressed in Christmas greens and filled with their Christmas guests. "Can't you just see that grand big Christmas tree reaching up to touch the ceiling and making all the room pretty and good-smelling?" "Now supposing court set amongst all the Christmas trimming, how would the Judge look from behind the green vines and red berries and long red candles banked up here?" "No, he ain't got the whiskers to look like Santa Claus and his ways are too dignified. That's from having his mind full of the law, him acting dignified, I mean. But to come back to remembering the Christmas tree and all this room full of Christmas people—"

"Hush now," interrupted a visiting midwife from another county, "don't tell me you-all had a Christmas party right here in this courtroom? But if you done so, I shore want to hear all about it."

That was a signal for all the midwives to start talking at once. Their guest waved her hands to stop them. "Take your turns," she suggested, "and tell me one at a time so I can make sense out of it. This way it all turns to jabber and don't give me no meaning."

"Ain't time enough now to tell," said one of the midwives. "Any minute now our nurse will come in and the meeting will start."

"No she won't neither," explained Martha Jackson. "She promised me a private sitting before the meeting starts, to thrash out some business that's personal. She said for me to come in five minutes, after she got through talking with the doctor on the phone. I'm going now; and, if you don't use up too many words, you'll have time a-plenty to tell our visitor about the Christmas party."

After it was decided by lot who should have the privilege of telling it, the story got under way. "In Midwife Clubs all around over the country," the teller began, "they give some notice to Christmas and the nurses and the grannies give each other little presents. But this year our Midwife Club took notice of Christmas in a grand fashion. Our December meeting turned into a big Christmas party and baby contest for the colored mothers and babies in this county. So many folks took a part in helping to make it a nice occasion that we forgot a long time ago whose idea it was in the first place. Our nurse and the County Health Department took a big part. Other folks with offices in the court house helped. The welfare people had a hand in it. The Baptist and the Methodist Sunday Schools here in the county seat gave twenty-five dollars to buy fruit for the Christmas tree. The Health Office in Atlanta sent down a doctor woman to judge the baby contest. A lots of folks took an interest and helped out."

"Who did you let come to such a big occasion?" someone asked to keep the story going straight.

"Well, a few special white people got invites, but mostly the folks invited to the party were the colored mothers and babies who had come to the mother and child health clinics here in the county. Mostly us midwives calls them *our* babies, for we catch most all the colored babies in this county. And let me tell you, ain't no mother of any color died in childbed in this county in two years. You see how them nurses and clinics and things helps out in such matters to make birthing babies a safer thing."

"But to come back to the party" . . . one of her midwife friends reminded her.

"Yes, I was just coming to the invites. The nurse sent them out from the Health Office to the mothers, like she sends out notices to them about clinics and other health meetings. Nothing fancy, just penny postal cards. But most of the mothers put them away for keepsakes, because they never went to a party before where they got invites all wrote out and sent through the mail. Most all of them sent back answers to the nurse. Excuse me a minute and I'll see if the nurse will let me show you some of the letters and cards they wrote her about coming to the party."

In a minute she was back with a stack of replies to the Christmas invitations. "The only reasons they said they couldn't come," the story teller resumed, "was that they couldn't get no way to come, like this woman that says her two mules won't pull together:

DC+16 1944

Mises Hom yes mom i sure Does want my Baby to take a Part But Lisen mis Hom one of our mules is Wile as a Buck and the other one is Slow as a tapin and i Just cant Get no one to BrinG us i sure wood Be Glad to come in to mises Hom

Daisy Benton
Jackson Ga

"Or they had sickness in the family like this woman whose baby had the whooping cough."

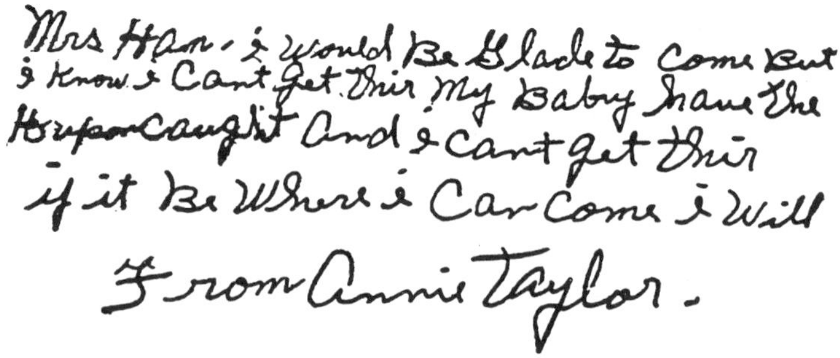
Mrs Hom. i would Be Glade to Come But i know i Cant get thir My Baby have the Hupercaught And i Cant get thir if it Be Where i Can Come i Will

From Annie Taylor.

"Mostly they just said they'd come if they could get a way to come. This card is that kind:

> Berner Ga
> Dec 14 1944
>
> I Recive your card and I Will try to Bring King Solomon if I can get away   Rosie Lee Lamar

"The mothers' share in the party was simply to get there, not no easy task for women with small children and living scattered about over the county. It fell to the rest of us to do the fixing up for the party. It took many a load of Christmas greens and berries and pot plants and things to dress up this big old courtroom to look partyfied. Us midwives that lived in the country caught rides into town so we could help. Sunday Schools and home people lent us trimming for the Christmas tree. And lots of people helped out different ways.

"One thing that took a lot of work was the big Christmas stockings, dozens and dozens of them made out of cotton mesh in different bright colors. They had to be cut out and sewed and filled with fruit. Martha finished filling the stockings the day before the party, after the rest of us had to go home. She thought they looked better full to brim. So she emptied out the stockings and stuffed the heels and toes with scraps of catalog paper and filled them up again.

"Late that night the nurse took one last look around before she went home. She noticed how stiff and tight the stockings were filled. She looked into the matter, then worked till nearly morning emptying more than two hundred stockings and filling them up again. The janitor told me she got three big waste baskets full of paper out of them heels and toes. She never said nothing about it, not wanting to hurt Martha's feelings."

"Do hurry and get folks to the party." One of the midwives prodded her to get on faster with the story.

"Yes'm, they're just starting to come now. The printed programs said nine-thirty in the morning was the time for the party, but it started soon as the first mothers and babies got there. Our nurse's secretary sat by the door of the party room and registered the mothers and their babies when they came in. Some of the mothers were right young girls, some were older women with big families, though they brought just the least ones with them. Then mothers of all ages in between.

"The babies got their names put down for the baby contest in three different bunches. There were the lap babies that couldn't even crawl and had to be carried in arms. Then there were the knee babies that could crawl about and pull up to stand by holding on their mothers' knees. Last of all were the yard babies that could run about on their own feet and play in the yard with the bigger children. All told there were a hundred and fifty babies and their mothers come to the party.

"As folks came in they scattered about over the room to visit and talk about their babies or to sit still and glory in the Christmas tree trimmed with shining lights and pretty things. With gold colored balls of fruit at the foot of the tree and the gay colored stockings of fruit piled behind the tree but not out of sight.

"When the program started, the president of our midwife club presided and we looked to the Lord first, like we do at a midwife meeting of whatever kind. An elderly white woman gave the Bible reading and the prayer. Then a scholar from the County Line Colored School welcomed the guests for the midwives and the Health Department. One of the young mothers gave an answer to the welcome on the part of all the mothers.

"About that time the white doctor that works with our clinics came in. He was not put down on the program, but our president knowed the mothers would want him to talk to them at their party. So he spoke a few words. Mostly he bragged on the mothers for trying to help the county and the state make all the people's health better. He bragged on them for keeping themselves well so they could take good care of their babies and others in the family. He mentioned how well their babies looked, how quiet and contented, letting their mothers enjoy the party. Then he bragged on them for the way their babies were dressed in good, substantial clothes washed and ironed nice, not in cheap finery nor dirty things. He said they showed nice care and good judgment in other things besides health.

"Then came the baby contest. The mothers and their babies went out one bunch at a time—the lap babies first. The doctor woman from Atlanta and our nurse went out with them. Us midwives were made welcome to go, but just our president went. Looking about for somebody to preside for her, she laid the honor on the nurse that presides over all the health in this whole part of Georgia. The nurse was proud of the honor, and she got the party crowd to singing our old songs. Different mothers took turns leading the singing while the nurse held each one's baby. They sang 'Down by the Riverside,' 'Golden Slippers,' 'When the Saints Go Marching In' and a lot of old favorites.

"When one bunch of babies came back another went out. When that was over, the nurse told what baby got the prize in each bunch and she explained how they chose the babies by their records in the clinics and by their condition of health. So the prizes belonged to the babies whose mothers had made the best efforts in the interest of their health.

"When that was over, some scholars of the Colored County High School came in to take their part on the program. In a big choir and in smaller arrangements of people they sang songs of Christmas time. The last and the one we all liked the best was one they sang special for the babies. They called it 'Lullaby on Christmas Eve.' The girl that sang the solo part had a voice like the mother of God singing her baby Jesus to sleep. One little child on the front row looked up at the choir and said, 'Sing that again for me.' And they did.

"The choir brought along a little first grade boy to give the salute to the flag. With his eyes on the Christmas tree, he forgot the words and had to be whispered to from behind.

"Their principal made a fine speech explaining about

the four freedoms. He added on another one—freedom from shame—but he didn't explain that. After his speech the school people had to leave. So the nurse gave them their golden balls of fruit from under the Christmas tree.

"The presiding midwife took the floor again to say how grand the occasion. 'That's all on the printed paper,' she said, 'but us midwives have got a little more to add.' Then we all, except that Martha wasn't at the party, bunched together and sang something we had arranged ourselves. After the first verse, the mothers joined in to sing with us. It went like this:

Mothers, get your business right
Mothers, get your business right
The Lord done told me to tell you
Get your business right

2. Sisters (midwives), get your business right, etc.
3. Nurses, get your business right, etc.
4. Everybody, get your business right, etc.

After our special singing was a prayer more specially for our babies.

"For the Lord's sake," her friends hurried her, "do get them stockings passed around. The nurse and Martha have about wound up their business and are standing up to come in here and start the meeting."

"Well, I'll hurry along now," the narrator said to their visitor, "and add the details and particulars for you when I got more time. I could tell all day about how the babies acted over them big stockings full of apples and oranges and tangerines and bunch raisins. And little surprises of paper dolls, and ends of ribbons, and teeniny toys and things in the stockings for the babies old enough to notice. The yard babies had the most fun. The mothers fixed their own and the lap babies' stocking of Christmas treat to take home. While things were still going big, a man came to take pictures and so the party folks moved down to the courthouse yard to have their pictures made. After that the party crowd scattered about over town to buy Christmas things, to visit around the square, or just to enjoy being in town the week before Christmas.

"Us midwives stayed on to talk over the party with the nurses and to get our presents off the Christmas tree where they had passed for decorations. Our nurse showed us a big table in the storeroom with apple Santa Clauses for the white well baby clinic and health party the next day. She said she would tell us all about that afterward. And she gave each one of us an apple Santa Claus too for a pattern to make some for our grands and great grands. And so our Christmas party was over in the courtroom but not in people's remembrance."

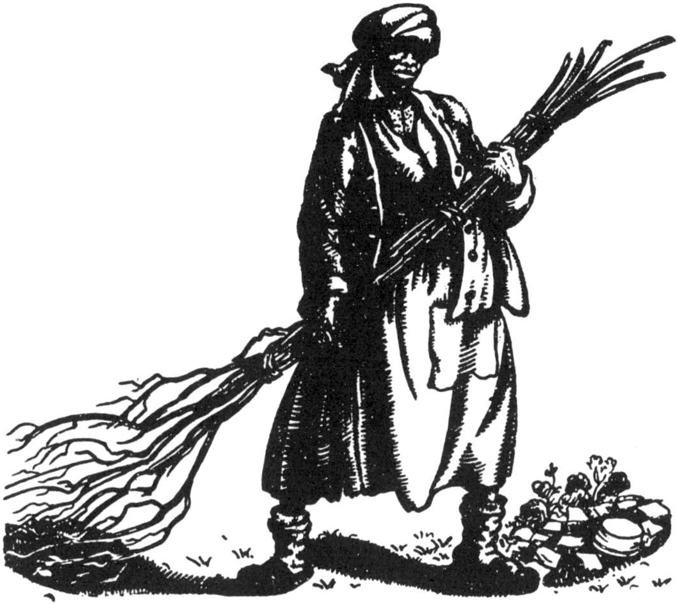

Visiting a Midwife at Home

"LET'S go out to see Martha Jackson, one of my midwives," said the county nurse, after the big Christmas party for midwives was over. "She was deeply worried about something yesterday—just what I don't know—and I think a visit would give her the cheering up she needs. Anyhow I need to talk with her about some prenatals coming in for the clinic this week." So another nurse and I bundled into the county nurse's car with Martha Jackson's gifts from the party Christmas tree and set out for her home eight miles out in the country from the county seat. The county nurse boasted that her car ran better on red clay roads than on surfaced highways. But even so, we got stuck and had to walk the last mile to Martha's house.

She saw us as we left the road and turned into her lane and she came eagerly down to meet us, exclaiming all the while about how happy she was to have visitors. Martha was dressed in some indescribable fantastic garb with two socks of two different colors on each leg and a fancy turban wound up out of two woolen scarfs and a kitchen towel. "These fancy clothes are my yard-cleaning outfit," she explained. Her big front yard showed the marks of the yard broom made of small branches with twigs left on. The yard was full of rose bushes and other shrubbery which had been freshly dug around. Flower beds bordered with old bottles showed signs of containing blooming annuals in season. Of all the dozens of colored midwives I have visited I have yet to see one who did not have flowers growing somehow, somewhere, about her place.

Patting her nurse affectionately on the back, Martha took us into the house, an unpainted frame house with a cotton field at one side and at the back, and piney woods stretching away at the other side. There were five rooms and a hall with a stairs to the attic running up from the hall. The house was better than some rural midwives' homes in that the interior was ceiled and there were windows throughout the house instead of the wooden shutters only, which make some houses so dark in winter when the shutters must be closed. Martha's house was beautifully clean throughout. The bed coverings were fresh and clean, the window curtains were newly laundered, and the bare pine floors were scrubbed white. In the hallway and front bedroom was a large display of hobnail glassware—evidently a family treasure. The house was rather crowded with furniture; because, as Martha explained, her widowed daughter had recently come home to live with her.

The sound of the daughter churning with an old-fashioned wooden dasher churn came from the kitchen. The smell of collards cooking for supper also floated in from that direction. The daughter, a good-looking, middle-aged woman, came into the living room soon with wood to mend the smoldering fire on the hearth. Her mother introduced her, telling us that this daughter was fifty, only fourteen years younger than Martha herself. Flora, the daughter, excused herself from joining us by saying she couldn't leave things in the kitchen just then.

Two little boys ten or twelve years old came shyly in from the back yard to have a peek at the visitors. Martha introduced them and they spoke politely and then poked each other and burst into giggles. When Martha asked where her husband, Tom, was, they said he was in the barn mending the mules' collars so he could hitch them to the wagon to haul corn the next day. They went to tell him about the visitors and to help him try to get the nurse's car unstuck. Martha told us that the larger of the two boys was her great grandchild, the other her daughter Flora's gift child that they were raising. Many a midwife's home has a gift child; that is, a child unrelated to the family and whom they have taken in because it has been orphaned by death or abandonment and has no other home. Martha laughed about the mischief the two little boys in her family could contrive together. She pointed to a leather strap hanging by the fireplace, and said she kept that handy to tend to the little boys if they got too rowdy after they went to bed at night.

The mended fire blazed up and soon had us backing off from it as we told Martha about the midwife Christmas party. The day before, she had caught a ride with someone working in town and had spent the entire day helping get ready for the party, helping to trim the tree and to fill the bright colored stockings. She inquired particularly if one of the doctors had got a stocking which he asked her to fill for him. Martha couldn't go to the party herself because this was the day she was expecting one of her patients to call her—but as yet the call hadn't come. The gifts we brought Martha from the party were simple, inexpensive things which the nurses and some of the visitors had brought for the midwives. The simple gifts were lifted far above their value by Martha's joy and appreciation. She teased the county nurse about the box of stationery, saying the nurse thought only penny postals were legal mail from the midwives. The apple blossom soap especially delighted her—and all the gifts she kept in her lap, touching them fondly now and then as she talked.

As professional women so often do when visiting, Martha and the nurses talked shop a great deal. The county nurse and Martha talked about prenatal patients coming to the public health clinics and others who should come. The knowledge and influence of the granny-midwives are a valuable asset to the public health program. Not only do the midwives know a great many people well but often they also have more influence with families they serve than the nurses do, when it comes to getting people to do things, especially *new* things, pertaining to health.

The county nurse mentioned one woman, one of Martha's neighbors, who didn't want to come to the prenatal clinic because she wanted to keep her secret longer. Martha laughed at the idea and said she could tell when a woman was two weeks pregnant because she "just looks indifferent to what she do at other times." She said once in a while some woman asked her for a remedy which would bring on an abortion. In that case she told the prospective mother to dig black haw roots in the woods and make strong tea and drink lots of it. "I tell her it will help her," said Martha, "and it do but not the way she thinks it will. Though I don't tell her then, it will make her baby hold on tighter and wait till the right time to get born."

Then Martha told about two cases she had recently cared for. "I do gorminate [abominate] dirty and nasty people," she began, "though I don't scorn nobody. This month I waited on a woman so nasty—excuse an ugly word, but *dirty* ain't strong enough. When I got there, not one clean thing about the place. I had to wash my hands in a battered old lard bucket—not no wash pan. No nothing. No wood even. I had to chop some wood before I could heat water to wash my hands. The man, after he got me there, never asked if he could do nothing, just crawled back in bed and snored till he shook the chimney.

"No sheet on the bed. The woman said she took the sheets off and never got them washed. I knowed she never had none. Her house and her family was always like that, sick or well. I had to put on her bed the big white sheet I carry in my bag to make a clean cover for work space. I had to spread out my white bag lining to work on. I got my sheet back, though, last day I went to tend her and the baby. It wasn't a pre-born baby but she never had nothing ready, though I had been there before and told her what to fix. Nothing ready for the baby except a fancy name. . . . The man makes right good wages, too, but they never try to have nothing. The mother lying in with a filthy old dress on. But I lived through it and the mother and baby did too—thank the good Lord!

"About the time I got the baby wrapped up in a piece of old blanket the other children started crawling out of the other room beds. Little white children they were, but so black with dirt you wouldn't know it. The oldest girl, about fourteen, started to scramble about making breakfast. And I just heated some water and washed up the whole lot of the children.

"After that I went back every day to tend the mother

and the baby. I showed the oldest girl how to bathe and take care of the baby. By that time they had got some clothes for it. Gradually she caught on and started to clean up herself, and then the whole place, and I helped her. If anybody took any interest to help her, I do believe she'd make a nice girl. No, they didn't pay me. I asked the man and he said, 'This baby ain't cost you nothing, has it?' I don't scorn nobody, but I do hate dirt and nastiness.

"Now let me tell you how far another woman went the opposite way. I showed her what to get ready and she done that and more too. When I got to her home, she had two white sheets on the bed and all the other bed dressings white. In the dresser drawer she had clean white towels and rags. And she was lying up in the bed with a white nightgown on and a white towel pinned around her head. She is real dark skinned and with all that white around her she looked like a big black wolf lying there. I said to her in fun, 'You look like a big old black wolf in the middle of all that white stuff.'

"She laughed at herself and said, 'You ain't so pretty nor white yourself, but I sure feel glad to see you.'

"Recently in November I stayed a whole month in Atlanta with a family who used to live in this county and got used to me taking care of the mother and the baby when babies come to their house. They had a doctor but they felt like they had to have me stay there. That kind of white family pays me more than any others and are nice to work with, though I don't get to count the baby among the ones I caught. The doctor puts it on his birth list.

"Seems like the fewer the doctors get with going off to war, the more the babies. I had to be away from home so much my daughter came to stay and look after her papa and the boys and things."

Just as the little boys announced that our car was unstuck, and we were getting ready to leave, a lame old colored woman came hobbling in. "This is Tom's old aunty," Martha said as we saw her coming. "Don't think no harm if she asks a million questions. She lives across the woods but she knows when we got company and comes over. She gets too lonesome to hardly live."

But, no, Aunt Tommy hadn't come just to see the visitors. She came to say Ticket Jones stopped by her house about noon to say his wife needed Martha and would Aunt Tommy come tell her. Aunt Tommy hadn't come sooner because she thought Martha was in town at the party. So Martha flew to change her clothes, grab her midwife bag, and catch a ride with us on her way to deliver another heir for Ticket Jones.

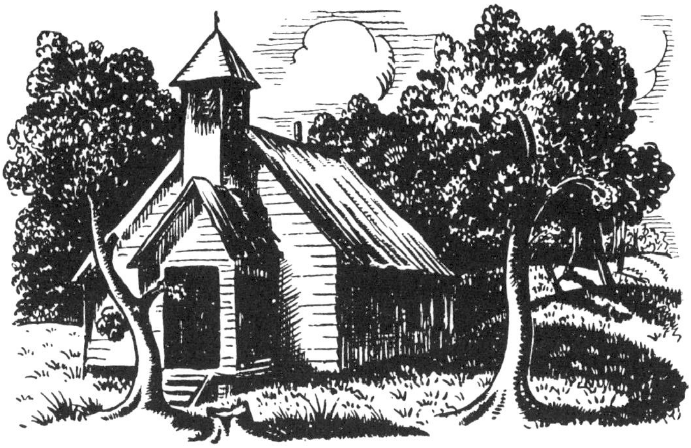

Aunt Jeanie Steps Down

When the granny-midwives talk about "stepping down off the Board," they mean retiring from practice when in good standing with health authorities. From time to time midwives are retired by the Health Department for reasons of old age or ill health, which make them unable to carry on their work. In Georgia they give up their licenses when they retire and promise on oath not to practice any more. Usually old age assistance is secured for them, to replace whatever small income they may have had from their patients. The old age pension is small, but is paid regularly and they can depend on it, which is more than can be said for their income from midwifery. Often the total amount for the year of old age assistance is greater than the annual income from their practice ever was. Since this financial help has been available, health authorities find it easier to retire old grannies who should be persuaded to quit. Sometimes considerable persuasion is necessary, for the grannies like their work and do not want to quit. Then too, they feel they are called of the Lord to do this work and final release from their duties must come from Him. Over and over the public health nurse hears from some old midwife too feeble or with eyesight too dim for her to be a safe attendant at delivery, "My mind ain't told me. The Lord ain't viewed me to quit."

Southern states have various ways of recognizing these faithful colored women's honorable discharge from active duty. The State Department of Public Health in Georgia gives a purple ribbon badge with the seal of the State of Georgia, the title of the State Department of Public Health, and the words RETIRED MIDWIFE in gold lettering. The pin attached to the badge bears the name of the midwife. These badges are awarded rather than a certificate of retirement, because any paper with the appearance of a legal document is likely to be mistaken for license to continue practicing. Usually the retirement ceremony and the awarding of the badge take place at a meeting of the Midwife Club, more often in May at licensing time. There may be a few guests, personal friends of the retiring midwife or visitors from the Health Department. The midwives who retire are encouraged to continue attendance at their Midwife Club, and they do when they are able.

Usually the retirement is as simple as that. But Aunt Jeanie's retirement service was neither usual or simple. Aunt Jeanie was nearing eighty, she had grown so feeble she had to walk with a stick, and her eyesight was failing. No longer was she a safe person to go on a delivery. She scorned the help of a younger and stronger midwife as unnecessary. When the public health nurse who supervised Aunt Jeanie's Midwife Club pointed out her infirmities, Aunt Jeanie simply said she couldn't retire because the Lord hadn't viewed her to quit. So the nurse and other members of the local Health Department were up against it. They couldn't take Aunt Jeanie's license by force and forbid her to practice. That would disgrace Aunt Jeanie in her own sight and in the eyes of her community. She was so tied into the life and the affections of the whole community where she had always lived that any mistreatment of Aunt Jeanie would incur the ill-favor of the whole neighborhood, even though they themselves may have seemed indifferent to her services. She was a member of a colored family long respected by white and colored people who knew them. She was a social leader among her people, a pillar in her church.

Perhaps one more talk with Aunt Jeanie would persuade her. But, no, the same answer, "The Lord ain't viewed me to quit." Something had to be done before Aunt Jeanie in her feeble state lost a case and brought tragedy where a stronger, clear-sighted midwife would have managed normally. "I can't have that half blind old soul called out in the middle of the night to risk her own health and possibly the life of a mother," the nurse pondered. "We'll have to think of some way to persuade her and to let people know they are not to call her any more."

Perhaps a special service for Aunt Jeanie at her church would do it. So the nurse talked with other members of the Health Department, with the minister of Aunt Jeanie's church, with colored and white citizens who knew Aunt Jeanie well. Everybody was eager to help, so preparation for the occasion got under way. Aunt Jeanie's sisters in the church scrubbed and cleaned and decorated the church. They brought their lace curtains to hang at the windows to give the church a "company look." They brought flowers from everywhere. Some woman brought an easy chair from her home to replace the short pew where Aunt Jeanie always sat in church. The chair was filled with fancy cushions and decorated with flowers. The whole neighborhood was fairly bursting with the secret. One little girl who stopped at Aunt Jeanie's house on some errand almost gave things away by asking Aunt Jeanie if she were going to church the next Sunday. "Hush your mouth, child," was the impatient answer. "Don't I always go to church? I don't need nobody to ask me do I aim to go to church."

Aunt Jeanie did go to church that Sunday, but she was late. As they waited for her, people remembered that she was usually late to every occasion except a birthing. She got there on time. Finally she came hobbling down the road with her stick. She was dressed in her best with a white collar and white gloves. A foolish little purple hat with an ostrich plume perched on her white hair. As always she carried her little midwife bag lest she be called on a case while at church and be caught unprepared.

As the usher led her up the aisle of the crowded church, the congregation stood to sing "When the Saints Come Marching In." When they were again seated, the minister rose to say that this service was dedicated to Aunt Jeanie in token of appreciation for her long years of service. They wanted to do her this honor while she was yet living and could enjoy it.

The minister took his Bible reading from the first chapter of Exodus, where the King of Egypt called two of the Hebrew midwives to him and commanded them and all the midwives to kill all the boy babies born to Hebrew mothers. "But the midwives feared God, and did not as the King of Egypt commanded them, but saved the men children alive." From his text, "But the midwives feared God" he derived his sermon, which soon became a personalized account of Aunt Jeanie's God-fearing life of good works. The sermon ended in this way: "And when she has laid down her work on earth and rested a while from her labors, then will come a day when the sweet golden chariot will swing low, down by her bedside, and carry her up to the pearly gates of Paradise. Then they will get out the record book where her name is writ in the blood of the Lamb and all the deeds she done. And St. Peter will start to ask, 'Did you let that little black baby die when his mama birthed him? Did you tend that little white child good when he was bad sick? Have you done what your nurse told you was the best way to do? Did you let any little baby go blind without no drops in his eyes? Have you everly been all times purity clean?' "

His sermon took on a lyric rhythm; and, when the questions began, Aunt Jeanie responded, as she no doubt would at the gates of heaven. So the last part of the sermon became an antiphonal chant between the minister and Aunt Jeanie. It was strangely moving and many of the congregation wept softly. The choir took up the singing of "Swing Low, Sweet Chariot" and "My Name Is Written in the Blood," keeping the music so low that the voices of Aunt Jeanie and the minister were clearly audible.

When she had answered the last question, the minister chanted alone. "Then an angel sets her feet on the golden stairs and leads her to the throne where all is snowy white. Then she puts on the raiment of an angel and lays down her heartful of sorrow and sits on a foot stool at the feet of Jesus beneath the golden light of heaven where the wind blows soft from the mountains of rest."

Following the sermon, a local doctor who had always known Aunt Jeanie spoke of her work as a midwife and as a practical nurse for children, saying she had always been patient and kind, clean and careful. Now he thought she deserved a long rest to enjoy her old age among people who knew and respected her. The public health nurse who had taught and supervised Aunt Jeanie said that when she was ready to retire, when the Lord relieved her of her burden of work, an old age allowance and a retired midwife badge were ready for her. A young colored woman spoke of Aunt Jeanie's work in the church and her leadership among the colored people in her community. Then there was presented to Aunt Jeanie a purse made up by people whom she had delivered at birth or nursed when they were small children. The purse contained a little over three hundred dollars and a list of those giving to it. Aunt Jeanie was asked to receive the purse and to say a few words.

She rummaged in her bag and brought up her midwife license. Holding it out to the nurse, she said, "The Lord has this day viewed me to quit and step down off the Board and leave the work to them that's abler in mind and body. And now if you got my badge handy, just pin it on me in the face of this congregation that knows I been passing faithful and never quit till the Lord knowed I can't hardly get along, and He lifted all the burden He laid on me." Only then did Aunt Jeanie accept the purse with simple thanks.

The minister asked Aunt Jeanie to make the closing prayer. Most of it was inaudible, for the choir began to sing:

Can't hardly get along
Can't hardly get along
My dear Lord knows
I can't hardly get along.

The congregation took up the singing and drowned out the voice of Aunt Jeanie.

2. I gotta sing to get along
3. I gotta mourn to get along
4. I gotta pray to get along
5. I gotta down my knees to get along—

Repeating the first stanza, only the choir sang, and Aunt Jeanie's prayer could be heard. Evidently she was praying for better service to mothers and babies to succeed the care of the passing granny-wife.

". . . Give folks the minds to know and the strength to do, so they can manage for better ways of looking after their women folks when they birth their babies. Lord, look down and take care of all the mothers and babies. Take care of this whole peopled world. And, Lord, in all Your hurry don't forget to take care of Yourself."

Part Two

To Talk with Them Sociable

"Now don't use up too many words in the manner of explaining the nature of the Granny-midwives' profession and their connections with the Board and with their nurses," advised Aunt Jeanie in talking with me about this book. "You know and I know—anybody with sense and feelings knows—that to get real acquainted with folks you got to talk with them sociable, and the grannies ain't no exception. So you save some of your words in that book for the times when we just talk sociable. Like when we meet together and talk sociable around among one another or when in a private sitting of two persons—maybe three—the talk gets away from business and turns sociable and we get better acquainted each with the other."

According to Aunt Jeanie's suggestion, this section of the book is made up of story-sketches from the sociable conversation of the granny-midwives. Their stories are written in the informal rambling style of their talking. An attempt to fit them into any short story pattern would take from the reader something of his chance to "talk with the grannies sociable," and thus get better acquainted with them and the people they know.

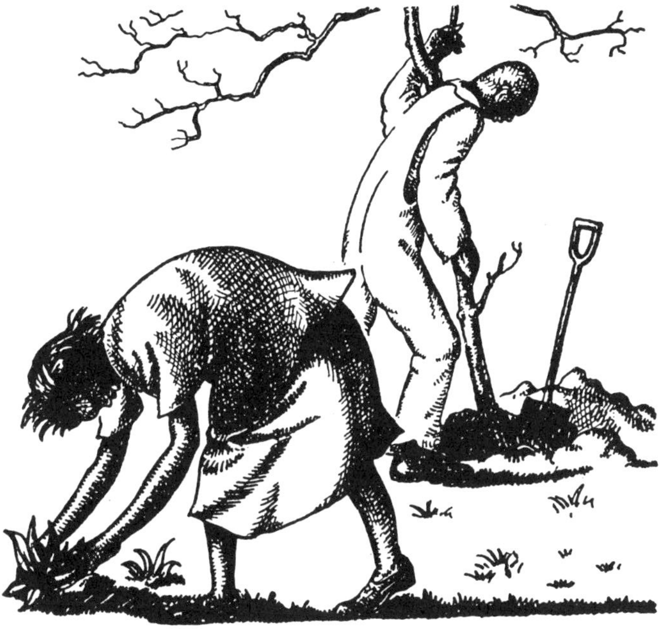

Then I Finds My Child

A SLIGHTLY bent little white-haired woman in a purple print dress and huge white apron looked in at Dr. Powell's waiting room door. Most people waiting there seemed to know her, for there was a chorus of "Come on in, Aunt Belle." "How are you, Aunt Belle?" "When did you get back from Carolina, Aunt Belle?"

"Got home last night," said Aunt Belle, coming on

into the room, her white apron crackling with freshly laundered starch as she moved. "Will you-all excuse me please if I speaks to young Doc?" And she knocked on Dr. Powell's inner door. When he stuck his head out, she greeted him with, "I just come by, Doc, to tell you that grandbaby of yours is all well and pretty again. He was plenty well so I coulda come back last week but his mama said to me, 'Aunt Belle, you got him well for us. Now why don't you just stay another week and enjoy our well baby?' So I done that. . . ." Then they talked on for a few minutes. Nobody waiting seemed to mind the delay, for it was evident they knew Dr. Powell's daughter and were eager to hear of her and the year old baby whom Aunt Belle had been nursing through a critical illness.

As Aunt Belle started to go, Dr. Powell asked jokingly, "Did they remember to pay you, Aunt Belle?"

"Yes, sir, they paid me good. They gave me a hundred dollars and bought me a train ticket too. Now I got to go."

"Out on a delivery?" he asked touching the worn little black bag she carried.

"No, sir, Doc, I'm going down to Love Hobart's. Their baby is bad sick and they so nasty with things I got a clean sheet in this bag and some clean white rags to clean that baby up good. Sorry folks like that don't need no baby."

"I wonder why the Lord lets people like that have families," interrupted a woman who was waiting.

"Love Hobart done had that baby behind the Lord's

back. That's my notion," Aunt Belle answered as she left and Dr. Powell turned back to his patients.

When it was my turn, I asked, "Who is Aunt Belle anyway? Everybody seemed to know her."

He laughed, "Sure, everybody knows Aunt Belle. She's the best baby nurse around here, the best I ever knew. The sickest baby grows well and happy, the most high-tempered smiles and goos and gurgles when Aunt Belle takes charge of it. People with sick babies had rather see Aunt Belle than me, and I don't blame them. Aunt Belle is a first rate midwife too. In her forty years practice she has never lost a mother—started by helping my father with confinement cases. Now let's get these bandages off this hand of yours."

A few days later I saw Aunt Belle again. In the early evening just after sundown I was walking in the colored section of town, a section that I like especially for its flowers. Flowering shrubs, perennials, annuals fill every yard. Even the most tumbledown shack has its array of varicolored zinnias and red and yellow four o'clocks. Now it was late November, the last chrysanthemums looked bedraggled and most annuals had given up blooming for this year. But the street was full of the laughter and commotion of children home from school and grownups home from work all collected in for supper. So I walked on much farther than ever before till I came to the end of the street. Way beyond the end of the street and away from any house was what appeared to be a huge old flower garden that had been allowed its own freedom to grow as it pleased.

But as I went nearer, a little brown house peeped out of the shrubbery like a perky brown wren peering out from her nest.

And there in the side yard near the fence was Aunt Belle cutting some late roses and piling them into her apron caught up to make a basket.

"Come in, lady," she invited. "I remember I saw you in young Doc's office. Come on in and see my granny flowers."

"Granny flowers," I thought, "which kind can that be?" as I walked around among a profusion of every kind of shrub, bush, or perennial that grows and blooms in the lower South. Tall crepe myrtles stretched above the roof at the back, wisteria dripped from the branches of an old tree, delicate coral vine festooned one of the old stone chimneys. Roses, sweet shrub, golden bells, pomegranates, flowering peach—something in bloom the year round. The cape jasmine was offering its last snowy blossom but already there were two camellia blossoms out and buds promising an abundance of them later in the winter. There were a few sprigs of early bloom on the kiss-me-at-the-gate, and the earliest blooming bulbs were pushing sturdy green tips through the earth. I wanted to see this wonderful garden in spring at the height of the blooming season. Well, I have seen Aunt Belle's garden in the spring and sometime I must tell you about it, but that is not what I set out to tell you this time.

"I picked these flowers for a birthday party," Aunt Belle explained as she came around the house to join me. "One of my babies has a party tomorrow when she is sixteen years old. You like my granny flowers? I calls them that because I plant something more in my garden everytime I am granny-midwife for a woman and catches her baby for her. All these years that makes a lots of granny flowers, for I caught a lots of babies. Come in the house and see my babies.'

I have no remembrance from that visit of what the house looked like inside. I remember only one whole corner filled with photographs of babies. A few were expensive, beautiful photographs, the rest were amateur snapshots, or the 3-for-10¢-while-you-wait kind. Pictures of babies born more than forty years ago, pictures of babies born this year; white babies, more numerous black babies; as Mam Bob once said, "babies of every kind and color."

"Two hundred and four of them," counted Aunt Belle, "all my babies that I help their mothers birth into this world. And some of them has grandbabies of their own now."

"You must have grandchildren yourself, Aunt Belle," I blundered. "Which pictures are they?"

"No, I don't have no grandbabies—I don't have no picture of my own little baby I lost and I never did see it."

Then as I started to go Aunt Belle laid her hand on my sleeve. "I ain't talked for years about it to nobody but if you wants to hear, I'd love to tell you about my lost little baby." I did want to hear.

"I was a gift child myself and was raised with folks

that weren't my kinpeople. They treated me good enough but my heart always reached out, even when I was a little bit of a thing, for folks that belonged to me.

"When I married with John Luke, I told him I wanted a whole cowpen full of little black children. He laughed at me and said to me, 'Go ahead, honey, and have all the babies you wants. I'll feed them and make little shoes for their feet.' John Luke worked in his shoe cobbler shop. His folks been good shoe cobblers way back yonder and John Luke had good trade. He was a thoroughly good man and everly a loving husband.

"But my babies didn't come and they did't come and the years passed by. Twelve years since I married with John Luke and I was past thirty years old. Then after all the years, I got in a condition and the women folks started telling me how bad it was to have your first baby when you are thirty. Some of them had grand-babies when they were that old. They teased me and said I aimed to skip a generation and birth my own grand-babies. The teasing made no never mind with me but when they kept saying I would likely die birthing my baby, I got scared and told John Luke.

"And he took some money out of his pocket and said, 'Don't fool with them old women's tales. You go ask Doc Powell what to do.' Neither John Luke nor me ever been to a doctor before in our lives. But I went that time. Old Doc Powell said plenty women had their first babies late in life and he told me what to do. And John Luke listened and he done all the hard work after that and was real gentle with me.

"He watched me sew clothes for the baby and he got some fine thin leather and made some little shoes for it and he said, 'I told you I'd make little shoes for your babies.' I planted more flowers for it to walk among and John Luke set out a chinaberry tree that grows big fast for it to climb and make swings on. If it was a boy I picked out John Luke for a name and if it was a girl he picked out Clarabelle for a name. And in two more months it would get borned.

"Then John Luke died over his shoe cobbler tools when his heart quit working. And I took down with a long sickness that carried me out of this world. My little baby dropped from me and I didn't know nor see. The neighbors buried it by the side of John Luke. When I first started to come back to this world and be at myself I heard them saying, 'Poor Belle, John Luke gone and now she lost her little baby.'

"Them words stuck in my heart and mind, 'lost little baby,' and all I could think was I had to find my baby like any mother would when her children get losted. Soon as I could get about on my feet I started looking. Seemed like sometimes I could hear a crying down in the smilax swamp—a pretty hiding place for little children but full of danger. Folks said the crying was just water birds screaming, but to my ears it was my lost little baby. So I kept on looking.

"Then one day I got all tangled up in a twist of yellow jasmine vines and fell down and hurt myself. When I went back to my house all over blood, folks said behind my back, 'We got to do it. Someday she will go off and hurt herself bad.' So they took me to old Doc Powell and though they made a great mystery I knowed what they went about. They thought I was going crazy and they wanted old Doc to sign some papers to put me away with crazy folks.

"Old Doc said to them, 'You-all go down town and do up your loafing or your trading or whatever you got to do and leave Belle here. When I get through with all these patients I'll take care of Belle.' So they went and I waited till Doc got through and come out to talk with me. And he said, 'Now, Belle, you listen to me. You not going crazy and you not sick. You just about to lonesome to death without John Luke and the baby. Some women are not made to have babies. But I tell you how you can ease your heart about babies. I'm getting old and I need help with my baby cases. I'm thinking you'd make a good granny midwife and could help me when a baby is a'borning.'

"But grannies has to be old," I said to him, for I had never seen one young as I was.

" 'No, they don't have to be, though they mostly are old," he said. 'They needs to be clean and intelligent and patient and willing, and you are all those things.'

"But granny midwives always been called by the Lord, like preachers are," I remembered. "I'd have to find out does the Lord want me to."

" 'All right,' he agreed with me, 'you get things fixed with the Lord and I'll stop for you the next time I have a labor case.'

"The Lord told me to go right ahead, for He was

taking care of John Luke and my lost little baby for me. He said He could have told me that all along only I just kept hunting by myself and never asked Him and He seen my lost little baby anywheres about.

"So I went with old Doc the next time he got sent for by a woman in her misery. I tended with him and he told me and showed me what to do. After that I tended with him a lots of times. Then come a day when he said, 'Belle, you could do this by yourself when it's not a hard case. I'm old and I can't be every place. And you already better than a lots of granny midwives. So I'm going to tell folks to get you to catch their babies.'

"After that and all these years I holp women birth their babies. I caught a lots of babies when their mothers birthed them and I nursed other babies out of their sickness and sometimes folks that has a doctor to catch the baby has me to stay and take care of the baby and its mother after the birthing. Over forty years I been a granny midwife and no mother ever died with me. But I don't take the credit to myself. I always had the Lord and one or the other Doc Powells to call on in trouble. Sometimes the Lord just said to me, 'You better send for the doctor to help you out, Belle, I'm telling you tain't safe not to.' I always minded the Lord and the Doctors and I everly been all times purity clean.

"Now I'm old and bent over and sometimes when I get called in the nighttime, I says, 'Lord, I'm old and tired. Give me my long rest and let me come up there to stay with John Luke and the baby.' But the Lord He says, 'You ain't so old as you will be. I got work yet for you to do down there and I'll give you strength. Go long, now and do your job and I'll see to John Luke and your little baby you lost.' So I goes—and when I has another little baby in these old arms—be it black or white—then one more time I knows I find my child, my lost little baby."

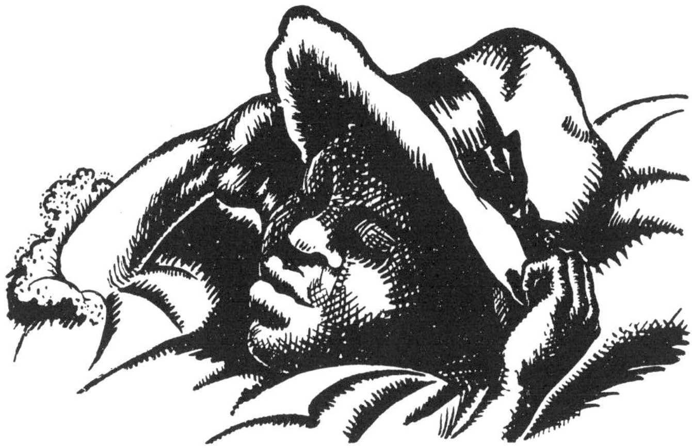

The Daddy's Hat

THE conversation had been running on old superstitions pertaining to childbirth and whether there was really anything in them. Some argued one way, some the other. Through all the argument Liddie Ruth Duffy had not said a word till some one finally turned to her and said, "Sister Duffy, what you think about old sayings? Do they work out to do good or harm or just nothing at all?"

Sister Duffy studied awhile and then she said, "Well now, anyway *one* time I knowed when an old saying worked out to do good way past what it was intended to do.

"You all remember Pinkie Paradise, that cute little baby girl I caught for Clotie and Larue Adams? Though now I'm talking about Pinkie a grown woman, not a baby girl. Well it's her that an old saying done good for, to my own knowing, for I knowed about it from start to finish.

"Pinkie was the baby of a big family and always been made a fuss over a lots. Her mama sent her to high school to get a good education out of books. But when I saw Pinkie prancing about acting foolish with the boys, I knowed she was studying some things not in the books. She fixed her hair in a high shiny pompadour, and she painted her mouth bright red, and she hung fancy earbobs in her ears, and she wore green shoes with her toes hanging out. And she laughed and danced and flirted her skirts and talked foolishness with the boys. Pinkie wasn't no bad girl—just young and careless and high-natured. Mostly she went with Roger Dell Bridges. He wasn't no bad boy—just young and careless and high-natured, like Pinkie.

"At the Fourth July mullet supper I saw them laughing and dancing and kissing and acting foolish—and I said to myself, 'Pinkie Paradise, you better keep them feet in them green shoes flat on the ground. Keep them feet flat on the ground or you gonna find yourself in a condition. Don't you listen to all Roger Dell's foolish soft talk. You keep your feet flat on the ground.'

"She did listen to the foolish soft talk and she didn't keep her feet flat on the ground. And first thing I know her mama, Clotie, come to see me and let out the news that Pinkie was in a condition and would I talk with Azelene Bridges about letting her boy Roger Dell marry with Pinkie. Clotie thought I would have influence with Azelene, seeing as we were sisters in the African Methodist Church.

"Roger Dell had owned up what us folks already knew, that Pinkie's baby was his'n. But his mama wouldn't let him marry her. Everybody knew—everybody but the school teacher herself—that Roger Dell's mama aimed to marry him off to a good-looking school teacher named Odessa Hightower. Folks laughed how Roger Dell's mama courted Odessa for him, asking her to fine suppers she cooked and sending her flowers to the schoolhouse. Folks said Sister Azelene tried to make her children marry above theirselves. Roger Dell never took much interest in the school teacher till he got Pinkie in trouble and then he turned toward the school teacher for excuse not to marry with Pinkie.

"But I told Clotie I was a granny-midwife and not no matchmaker. Anyhow I wouldn't want my girl to marry with somebody that didn't want her. And Clotie said now she had studied on it she didn't either want her girl to marry Roger Dell if he didn't want to marry her. She said her and Larue would take care of Pinkie and the baby and some day she would marry somebody a lots better than Roger Dell Bridges. Then she engaged me to wait on Pinkie when the time come.

"So I was there, and Pinkie had a hard time. She was little and young but she never made much noise. Mothers not married to their baby's daddy act more quiet than others do that got a husband waiting around. Girls not married ain't got nobody to put on a show for. Pinkie had a bad time but she never made a big fuss. I loved Pinkie a heap and I wanted to do all in my power. After a while I thought of an old saying that if the mother puts on a hat of the daddy of her baby and pulls down on the brim it makes the pains do more work and the baby get borned. It wouldn't do no harm to try. So I made up my mind to go to Sister Azelene's and get Roger Dell's hat for Pinkie.

"I left Clotie to watch Pinkie and went down the road a long mile to Sister Azelene's house. It wasn't sunup yet but a thin twist of smoke was rising up from the chimney and the lamp was lit. She come to the door and I didn't set down for a polite visit but went straight to my business.

"I asked for Roger Dell and she said he done gone off to work. I knowed better, for I could see through to the next room where he made a hump in the bed and where his pants laid across a chair. So I said, 'I know better. He's laying in there in the bed and little Pinkie Paradise having his baby. Bad enough for a woman to bear her pains for a man that she's snoring in the face of every night but to bear them for a man that's running after a school teacher his mama picked out and this minute laying up in his warm bed sleeping while his mama that's my sister in the church stands here before the Almighty and me and says he's gone off to work. That's a poison lie if I do say it to your face, Azelene Bridges. . . . But I ain't asking you to let Roger Dell marry Pinkie. She's too good for him. I just wants his old hat for Pinkie to wear in the bed to pick up her pains and get this baby of Roger Dell's borned fore it kills her and your boy has one more sin on his soul.

" 'Don't stand in my own house and call me a liar,' " his mama screeched. 'And I ain't give you no hat.'

"Then I saw Roger Dell's hat hanging on the dresser arm right there in the room, his Sunday hat. A fine pretty colored costly felt hat with a little green feather stuck in the striped ribbon band. I just grabbed that hat and left.

"His mama rared and charged, 'You can't take that hat,' she screeched. 'It cost Roger Dell eight dollars and it's his Sunday hat. You can't put that fine hat in no child bed with no Pinkie Paradise. How you think he feel?'

"It was more of a point how Pinkie feel. She'd feel better with that hat on her head. So I put the hat on Pinkie and it help her birth a fine boy, the spitting image of Roger Dell. Pinkie turned plumb crazy about that baby. After I got it washed and fixed she held it close and hardly wanted other folks to touch it. Clotie and Larue hung over the bed till Pinkie got worried with them and said, 'This is my baby. This is my baby all by myself.'

"Every day I went to tend Pinkie and wash the baby. On the seventh day, while I was washing the baby, somebody knocked on the door. Clotie was gone to the store and Larue gone off to work. So I gathered up the baby and went to the door. There stood Roger Dell. He said, 'I come by to get my hat.'

"I give him the hat and thank him kindly for the use of it and the help it give Pinkie to birth her baby.

"Then he said, 'That Pinkie's baby you got there?'

"And I said, 'This shore is Pinkie's baby I got here. And I reckon you know who else's baby this is besides Pinkie's.'

"He never said nothing. Just took up his Sunday hat and went off.

"Next day he come with a package. 'Got a cradle gift here for Pinkie's baby,' he said. 'Could you see does it fit?' I brought the baby to the front room and he put on its head a blue silk bonnet cap with ruffles and lace and little pink flowers. It fit good and looked pretty and I took it for Pinkie to see.

"Next day he stopped by to ask what was the baby's name. Never had no name yet. Every day he come. Asked could he hold the baby. Could he see Pinkie. Pinkie said she ain't let no man outside the family see her in the bed. She said it ain't nice to do that. He would have to wait till she was able to get up and dress herself.

"When he did get to see Pinkie, Roger Dell told her he wanted to marry her and the baby and he asked her would she. Pinkie said she'd have to study about it. And she asked him what about that school teacher. And he said, 'Nothing about that school teacher. She ain't had me no pretty little boy baby, did she?'

"Then Pinkie asked him, 'What your mama say?'

"And he said, 'This is my business I keep in my own mind and I ain't asked mama.'

"Pinkie still said she'd have to study about it.

"When she studied long enough to suit her mind she told Roger Dell her and the baby would marry him but she wanted a proper and pretty wedding in the church.

"Roger Dell's mama put in to say they better just go to the court house and get married quiet. If they have a wedding in the church, it would bring things to people's notice and they would start to gossip.

"Then Clotie she said, 'Folks that want to gossip done gossiped till they run out of gossip. What you thinking about? This baby Pinkie got ain't no military secret. Anyhow, Pinkie is my girl and the bride's mama helps fix for the wedding—not the man's mama. And I done fixed with the preacher for Pinkie to get married in the church.'

"After that Sister Azelene said they ought not to take the baby to the wedding. But Pinkie cried and said she wanted her baby at her wedding for a love token. And so they took the baby to the wedding and Clotie held him so Pinkie's dress wouldn't get mussed up. . . . But you folks know what a nice wedding and how pretty Pinkie looked and all the presents she got. And Roger Dell's mama spreading on and acting like the wedding was something she thought up herself.

"Pinkie and Roger Dell went to housekeeping over on Mr. Bob Hamilton's place. And Clotie and Azelene got as thick as two in a bed and wore a slick path across the field going back and forth to each other's houses to talk about their grandbaby. Then Roger Dell had to go off to war, and Pinkie and little Hatler Dell come back home to stay with Clotie and Larue.

"Now Pinkie is expecting again. She come over this week to engage me to wait on her when she births this baby. She laughed and told me that the last time Roger Dell was home before he got sent across to fight she told him she was in the family way again. And he took off his soldier hat and throwed it at her and said, 'I'll be off in the war and can't be here with you. But here's my hat to wear in the bed.'

"And she said to him, 'Watch out, Roger Dell, you remember the other time I wore a hat to birth my baby I got married to a man. You want me to do that again?'

"Then he snatched his hat back and laughed a lots and said to her, 'Pinkie Bridges, you birth this baby bareheaded. You hear me? You birth this baby while you stay bareheaded?' "

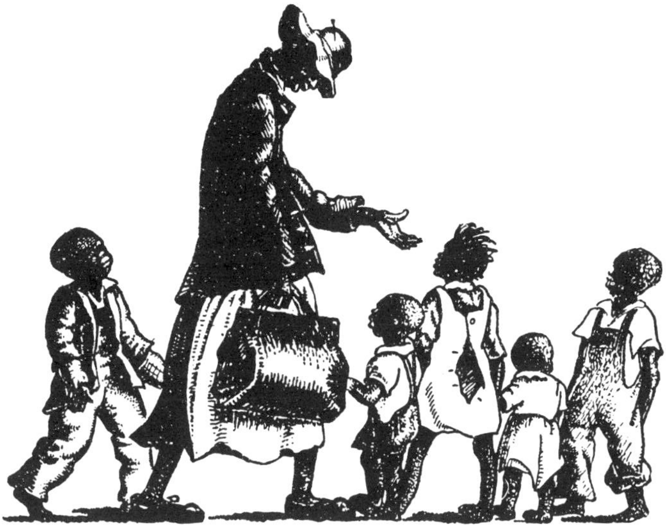

I Just Got a Touch with Children

On Friday we had a penciled penny postal from Aunt Rosella Simms which read, "A cumen in Sat to get Silva Knight lak to carry fren mete you Col Lady city up Noarth gesting wit me."

So we were not at all surprised to find Aunt Rosella and her colored lady guest from up North waiting when we arrived at the Public Health Office on Saturday morning. Before the county nurse could get the door unlocked, Aunt Rosella was introducing her guest. "I want you ladies to meet my friend, Sister Mandy Aikens. Sister Mandy used to practice with us other granny midwives in this county fore she went up north to live with her daughter Lillie Maude. That was fore you come here, nurse, so you wouldn't know.

"Proud to meet you," responded Sister Mandy. "Will you-all excuse me, please, for my rheumatism strings on my legs. They don't add no style to my looks but Sister Rosella said they wouldn't make no never mind to you ladies if they helped my health."

Both of Sister Mandy's ankles were bound with wide strings of red wool flannel tied in fancy bows. We settled ourselves to get acquainted with Sister Mandy as Aunt Rosella took up her story.

"Sister Mandy used to live on Mr. Tom Davis's place, ain't that right?"

"Yes'm, in that old house with the four chimneys and with the high fig bushes in the front yard. Go on, you tell, Sister Rosella."

"Well," Aunt Rosella continued, "after Sister Mandy's children got growed up out of the way, the Lord laid on her the burden of granny work. She was a good granny midwife and a lots of women in their misery sent for her. She was big and strong and kind-hearted and patient. And she had a touch with children. They loved her and done anything she wanted, though they might not mind their mamas so good. All the children called her Ma Mandy and the grown folks took up that name to call her. So's she got to be Ma Mandy to everybody that knowed her."

"They called me The Bringer too, the children did," Ma Mandy interrupted.

"So they did," Aunt Rosella went on. "I just hadn't got to that part yet. The children knowed when Ma Mandy took her little black bag and went to see a family there would be a little new baby in that family. So they called her The Bringer. When they would see her pass they would wonder whose mama she gonna bring a little baby. They would swing on the gate or run out to meet her and say, 'Who you carry a baby to this time? When you bring us a baby child?' Then a thing happened that broke down her practice, but you tell that part, Ma Mandy."

Then Ma Mandy took up the story. "I always done the best I could. Angels couldn't do no more. But one year, scattered over the country in a wide circle of trips, I caught three sets of twins. Just *three* sets it was for certain. But the story got bigger as it traveled from mouth to mouth and soon everybody knowed I brought ten sets of twins in one year. No use to argue it wasn't but three, for folks always rather believe the biggest tale. That story about ten sets of twins went round about—till folks got superstitious that if they sent for me they would shore get twin babies. Now folks likes twins after they get them but most people wouldn't reach out and bring down two babies at once on purpose if they could settle it beforehand.

"The colored folks where I had most of my work with said, 'Shore you get two babies at once if you send for Ma Mandy. Ain't the little children called her The Bringer? Ain't children knowing beyond their years in things grown folks can't see nor know? No, I don't want me no twins. And I ain't send for Ma Mandy no more.'

"The white folks tried to make out they went above superstitions. They said, 'Listen to them superstitious Negroes turning Ma Mandy down because she brought so many twins in one year. Thank the Lord we ain't like that.' But *they* never called me no more neither and my practice broke down."

"That was when you went to cook for Mis' Delia Davis, wasn't it now?" Aunt Rosella questioned to keep the story going.

"Yes'm," Ma Mandy remembered, "that was the time I cooked for Mis' Delia. They treated me nice but they had a grown-up family and my heart longed for little children. Then my daughter Lillie Maude took down bad sick and I went up North to tend her and I been up there going on six years."

"And how do you like your new home, Ma Mandy?" I asked, for it would never do to have the story end there.

"My daughter and her family live nice," Ma Mandy answered. "They all got good jobs and make good money. They moved to a more stylish part in the city since they get more money. Not so many colored people where they live now. Though I can't see no use to live next to white folks if they don't pay you no mind. Lillie Maude's children—all of them grown and got jobs—tries to tell me how it's worth a heap to have rights to live outside the part of town where everybody is colored folks. Young colored folks think a heap and talks a heap about their rights. Up North colored folks got a right to vote in elections and a right to set by white folks traveling. To young folks striving to rise up in the world, I reckon them rights mean a lots. But to me they turn out to be cold rights. Most of the white folks that talks about race equality just talking with their minds, their feelings ain't ready yet for them to make us equal with them I don't think. When I sit by a white person traveling they let me do it but I can feel how they feel inside themselves, 'Good gracious I'm sitting by an old Negro woman.' And they don't forget I'm a Negro and it ain't my privilege to forget it either.

"First time I got enough money I earned myself I come back to visit where folks knows me—black or white irregardless—and asks me how's my rheumatism and how is Lillie Maude and Caroline and the children. Some folks can live in a city and set on their rights and stay happy, but not an old woman like me that was raised sociable and always had a touch with children. Me, I couldn't never be satisfied to stay in a big city where folks is so crowded up and so cold and unspoken in their ways."

It was then that we found out really why Aunt Rosella had paid us this visit. The Silva Knight [silver nitrate] was only an excuse. What she really wanted was to get Ma Mandy's midwife license renewed so she could take up her profession again and live again with surroundings and people she was accustomed to. To help convince the nurse that she still had a touch with children Ma Mandy told us about her experience with a baby school [nursery school] in the city she had recently come from.

"Lonesome I was that day," she began her story of the baby school venture, "lonesome nearly 'bout past living. So I put on my hat and I got my pocket book and I left that big stacked up building where Lillie Maude lives with a lots of other colored families we don't know nothing about at all. I rode a long piece and then I walked a piece. After a time I saw a white lady herding a lots of little white children out of a little cooped up yard space into a building. It looked like a schoolhouse but they weren't big enough children to go to school—just past being babies they were. So I wandered in to see what sort of place it might be. A lady asked me what did I want and I was too plumb scared to have good mind. So I said I wanted a job. Then she went off to see what to do about me and I stepped down the halls towards a big room with a lot of commotion raising out of it. A white lady was trying to get a whole room full of little white children to lay down and take a nap. But they kept right on raising ruckus and wouldn't do it. They were shouting like a song, 'I won't take a nap! I won't go to sleep!' over and over they sung it loud as they could.

"I just stepped to the door and I says, 'I like to know how you-all gonna help yourselves. Little children always do what I wants them to do, and I wants you-all to go to sleep.'

" 'Big old black woman,' they said to me. 'Big old black woman, who you?'

" 'Little children used to call me The Bringer,' I said.

" 'What you bring us?' they asked me then.

" 'Sleep what I bring this time, but you-all can't have it till you get ready.' So they pulled off their little dresses and their little pants in a rush and kicked off their little shoes and jumped under their little blankets.

" 'Now let me see you bring sleep,' they said.

" 'Listen to you!' I said. 'You-all smart children and you know you can't *see* sleep coming. You got to *feel* sleep coming. Shut up your eyes and listen to me sing while I brings sleep.'

"What I sing to put children to sleep? Just what I makes up as I goes. That's the onliest way to sing to little children the right way. Just make up the song as you go. That time at the baby school I sung about how different little things go to sleep—little birds with their little heads under their wings, little cats stretched out long. . . .

"Well, fore anybody knowed it all them little children was soft asleep and me I went to sleep too. When we woke up the little children said, 'Look, our Bringer brings some sleep to herself, too.'

"I stayed around that baby school all that day till the mamas came and took their children away. And then the lady that runs the school and the ladies that help her said to me, 'How do you do it? Tell us how you do it.'

" 'Do what?' I says. Then they said to tell them how

I managed with little children so they were nice and behaved good. And I said they weren't nothing to explain. I just had a touch with children.

"Then they talked about how these children acted bad and had mind doctors working on them to find out why don't they be nice children and mind they mamas. And the mind doctors don't have no good success with these children. Then long comes a big old Negro woman and the little children all lamb out and turn good and behave so pretty. They say it was magic. But I say I ain't never done no conjure magic and ain't never had no faith in it. I just had a touch with children.

"Then they said would I come back the next day and see if it would turn out the same. I went back and the children were proud to see me and were good as pie all day. That evening the ladies said they would like to have me about and they would give me a job. Only they couldn't hire no Negro nor no woman who couldn't read to work with the children. That weren't allowed at all. Though they could hire me to work in the diet kitchen and keep out of the children's sight.

"But no matter how easy I slipped into that building, the children knowed I was there. They didn't have to *see* me come. They just knowed. And they wouldn't leave me be to cook and the grown folks that run things wouldn't have no unreading black woman on the work list with them. So I reckon the mamas and the people at the school went right on paying out big money to the mind doctors and worrying their own minds because their little children didn't be nice and act pretty. Ain't it a sight what trouble and bother and money some white folks will use up to keep their little children from growing up natural?"

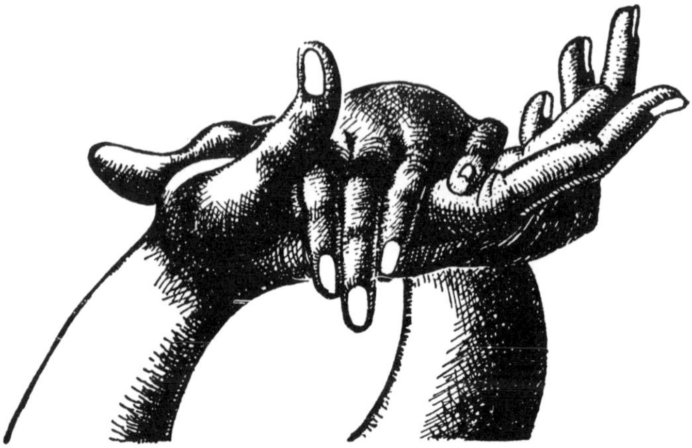

I Fairly Drink Up Kindness

AUNT LEE ANN LYONS carefully settled her white cotton feed sack of groceries outside the door before she spoke to us. Then she came in with her hands in her sweater pockets, carefully holding something. "Here, Nurse, honey, I brought you a present," as she held out six speckled guinea eggs, three in each hand. "My two old guinea hens are laying again, though I can't find one of them's nest. I put these in my pocket thinking I'd trade them for that much worth of fish hooks. The storekeeper's children where I trades likes guinea eggs. Then I had another think coming. I thought, 'Why don't I take them to my health nurse that helped me get the old age pension and done a lots of things for me?' Here they are, honey. I hope you likes guinea eggs."

"Indeed I do," answered the nurse. "I used to help my grandmother hunt the guinea hens' nests and take out the eggs with a spoon. Now what can I do for you, Aunt Lee Ann? Here, let me clear these papers off this chair so you can sit down."

"I didn't come to do no asking for myself," Aunt Lee Ann said, helping to clear the chairs of the clutter of reports the nurse and I were working on. "I stopped by to tell you that a white lady that lives two miles down the main road from my place is sick with having fall out spells, and I'd love for you to go out to her home to see her sometimes right soon if you can get off."

"Do you have any idea what's wrong with her?" the nurse questioned.

"She's expecting a baby—her first one—and she's been having these fall out spells. Her sister that stays there with her come after me yesterday when she was having one of them spells. I told the sick lady she ought to come up here to your pre-mother clinics but she said she knowed you'd mix her in with the colored folks—"

"But we always take the trouble to have separate clinics," the nurse interrupted Aunt Lee Ann.

"Yes'm I knowed it and I told her, but she wouldn't believe it was the truth. Her husband is in the war."

"Then the government will provide care for her and the baby."

"Yes'm, I told her that too, but she said there again

the people in charge of the government favored the Negroes so much she knowed they'd put her baby to sleep all mixed up with Negro babies and herself right in among the Negro mothers. I tried to tell her different, but she said what did an old Negro woman know about hospitals and the government's ways. And then she had another fall out spell. I'm scared she's gonna die if she don't get something done."

"Now sit down, Aunt Lee Ann, while I finish these reports and you get acquainted with my friend. Then I'll stop by to see her on my way out that road to see a t. b. patient that has just come back from Alto. You can ride out with us—unless," she added teasingly "you'd rather take the bus."

"Rather take the bus? Hush your mouth, honey. What you talking about? I dreads like murder to scrouge on a bus so full of folks they standing up all the way back. I has to wait to get on with the last and then I mashes folks flat squeezing me and my sack of rations through all the way to the back—and then squeezing back through to the front again just five miles down the road from town to where I get off. I never had to bother with no bus when I had Ida to come with me to town to carry our rations home."

It was not till Aunt Lee Ann sat down opposite me that I saw the great scar that covered one whole side of her face, almost closing one eye, distorting one ear, and extending on down to the shoulder. But what was lacking of beauty in her face was in her hands. Few hands that I have seen were so beautiful as hers—small and gentle like a woman's, sensitive and sure and strong like a surgeon's. I could not help exclaiming, "What beautiful hands!"

"You think my hands are pretty?" Aunt Lee Ann spread them out on my lap for me to see better, then drew them back shyly. "My husband always liked my hands. He was the first person in my life that ever found one thing pretty about me."

"Won't you tell me about him," I begged.

"I'd love to. My mama said I was a pretty baby to match the pretty name she gave me. Then when I was just starting to walk I fell in the fireplace and burned myself this way. My mama was a proud woman and she never could love me after my face turned so ugly. She didn't want folks to see me and ask was that her child. She kept me at home and she beat me for childish waywardness that for my pretty little sisters went unnoticed. When I got bigger she left me at home to mind her babies and the house.

"That way I never had none of the dressing up and the courting and funning that young girls belong to have in their time. But I learned to work good, to cook and do fine laundry and to tend babies.

"Then one time when I was just past seventeen a drummer came in a two-seated, two-horse buggy to show his goods to the stores in the part of the country where we lived. He took down sick and had to stay a week in that neighborhood. The elderly colored man driving for him had to stay too and he boarded at our house. He was the onliest person up to that time that was ever kind to me. The last day he was there mama got mad and beat me with a lightwood stick. He took the stick away from her and said he wanted to take me home with him and marry me. Mama said, 'Marry that ugly thing!' And he said, 'She don't look ugly to me. She's got beautiful hands and little feet, marks of a lady in any color.'

"Mama was glad to marry me to anybody and get me off her hands. And she thought Joe Lyons was a man of property because he was dressed nice and talked about living in a painted house. She gave me a snake's trail quilt and one of old Bessie's pups and a pair of new shoes that hurt her feet. And Joe Lyons, my husband that was to be, put them things and me on the back seat of the buggy and we drove off with the drummer to this town, long miles away from my home place. And we never went back to mama's no more.

"Joe bought me a new dress and a hat with a long veil. Then he got a courthouse license and had a preacher to marry us. I got the license hung up in my house for a picture on the wall. He said he wanted to marry me with the Law so his kin people nor nobody couldn't come in and take his house and ground from me after he was gone.

"Always he was every way kind to me. He gave me a good home and made a living for me. He took me with him places and he was always proud of my pretty hands and never thought me ugly. But he was an old man and he never done my nature no good. So we never had no babies. When my nature was strong there were times when I had thoughts of young men. But my thoughts were my own privacy and I stayed faithful to Joe.

"I wanted us to take some orphan children to raise but he was afraid he'd die and leave me to raise them by myself or he'd get feeble and be on my hands to tend besides the children. He worked beyond his years and strength to make a living. One evening after I'd been with him some twelve years he came in from work and I called him to supper. He said he wanted to stay out in the night-cool a little while and get rested. Then he sat down on the edge of the porch and died quiet—the way he lived.

"After that I raised five children and made a living for them. Not kin to me nor to each other, just orphan children without no home. They were great big children when I took them one after another, for I couldn't tend a little baby and work out on our own place and for other people to make a living. Before I hardly knowed it they were all grown and married and gone off up North to big cities to work where's the big money. They not good to remember and write me nor send me things. Maybe if I coulda taken them when they were little bitty things I coulda made me a close family with them. I don't know.

"Joe's Aunty that was getting too feeble to practice learned me how to be a granny-midwife and the nurse here learned me more better ways to tend women with babies. But I'm near seventy now and all alone since Ida left me. For the past ten years it's been just me and Ida there on the home place."

"Could you tell about Ida as we ride along?" the nurse broke into the story. "I'm ready to go now, Aunt Lee Ann."

As soon as we were settled in the car she was careful to give Aunt Lee Ann a chance to pick up her story again. "I always meant to ask you where Ida came from," she offered as a new starting point for the Ida story.

"White man had her for some years. But she wasn't a pretty creature and limped a little. She looked poor and sorry and bad. So he didn't treat her good nor want her no more. That's when I took her to my home with me. I fixed her good things to eat so she got nearly about fat. I doctored her sore leg till she could walk good. I pulled Spanish moss to make her bed soft under her blanket. And she got well and contented and had a good home with me.

"She was a great help to me and a heap of company too. Whatever I done except the housework Ida helped me do. It wasn't in her nature to do housework but in the outside work she done hardest or the heaviest part. Even when I went to the woods to pick blackberries or huckleberries or to hunt wild plums she went ahead and scared the snakes away. One time when we were tending cotton down by the river she got struck with lightning and fell over and lay there. But I revived her with buckets of water from the river and the next day she was able to work again.

"She went with me on long trips to catch babies and waited for me till I could come home again. She went with me to town to carry back our rations. Sometimes she grunted and groaned to herself but she never talked back, she never called me ugly, nor she never forgot me. She always woke up first in the morning and waited quiet till I woke up and spoke to her. Then she knowed I was up and we could eat breakfast.

"That last day before Ida died we had been pulling corn fodder all day and carrying it to the barn. Ida worked hard as I did and never a grunt nor a groan. We worked till coming dark and then come home. I fixed supper and gave Ida things she liked to eat—fresh green roasting ears cut up fine so she could eat it with her bad teeth. She had a good appetite. Once in the night I got up and went to see about Ida but she was all right.

"When I woke up the sun was shining high and it was late. I looked for Ida, but she wasn't there. I knowed something bad was wrong. So I jumped up and ran out of the house in my nightgown calling Ida. No nicker from Ida to answer me. And there she lay in her stall on her moss and her blanket cold and dead. She died in the night sudden and quiet. I had to hire somebody to haul her off to the woods and bury her. Since then I thought some about another mule, but I can't think it would ever work with me as good as Ida. So I lives alone without no work animal nor no man.

"My heart and mind always told me I'd rather be lonesome without Joe than to risk another man that maybe would think me ugly and not notice my pretty hands that Joe loved so much he never saw the rest of me ugly. And maybe no other man would be kind to me like Joe. And I couldn't stand that. I fairly drink up kindness."

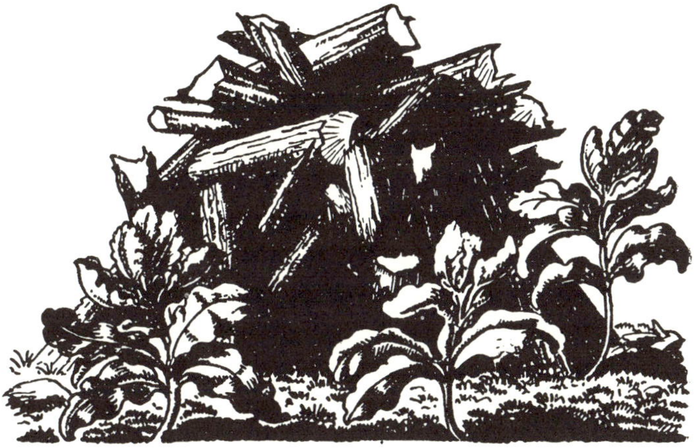

Too Many Kin People

AUNT ROSELLA's license to practice midwifery had been taken from her for serious violation of the regulations of the State Department of Health, and the other midwives in her county were discussing the situation with one another and with their supervising nurse.

"She listened to the kin people of her patients too much," Aunt Lula explained. "The worst things that goes against us midwives following the rules under the New Law are folks that won't try to be one bit clean and kin people butting in to do things their way. The mothers and the mothers-in-law are the worst to go contrary to what us midwives are supposed to do, though they mostly do things behind our backs. Not a midwife here but can testify to that." And they did testify to it.

"Just last week I told folks where they had a new baby not to give the baby nothing but boiled water—not no teas of no kind. And to give the mother of the baby plenty of a lots of different things to eat. Then when I went back, the mother was giving her girl just bread and coffee because she thought other things would make the girl sick. And she was dosing the baby with dried turtle heart tea to give it long life. All that going on behind my back." Aunt Molly would have testified further as to the iniquities of her patients' kin people, but someone interrupted her.

"And me, I told my last patient to stay in the bed nine days after she birthed her baby. I went back the third day and there she sat in the rocking chair, all dressed up and shelling peas for dinner. Her mother-in-law said she got her up out of the bed because Christ rose on the third day. Now I aim to be a good Christian and follow my Jesus, but I just don't see the connection there."

"Just too many kin people," Aunt Lula had her say again. "Too many kin people at a birthing. A lots of times women that claim to be kin crowd in the house and don't do nothing but sit underfoot and look on. And they sit out in the kitchen and burn up all the cook wood and tell dirty tales. Me and one other person is a plenty at such a place and time. . . . But now it's time to enter into the business of our meeting. Let the house come to order and sing 'I Shall Not Be Moved' to start our devotion before the business comes up."

After the business had been disposed of and the midwives had taken a slow departure, their nurse had a call to make on Martha Lee Owens, a young mother who was supposed to come home from the hospital that day. Since she lived out past Aunt Lee Ann's house, we picked up Aunt Lee Ann's mail. But she was not at home. "Probably out on a call with somebody who jerked her up without any notice," we guessed.

Following Aunt Lee Ann's directions, "You go down the road past my house to the first branch; then turn toward the north and go about a mile; and she lives in a red house trimmed with white," we arrived to find Aunt Lee Ann there folding freshly washed blankets and quilts and putting the last touches on Martha Lee's house, already in perfect order. Martha Lee wasn't coming till the next day.

"And it's a mercy she don't come till tomorrow," Aunt Lee Ann said as we helped her fold the last quilt. "Do sit down and let me tell you. Too many kin people that's what was the matter with this house.

"Now Ollie Owens, the man of this house, ain't got no kin people but the girl he married. He was raised an orphan by Mis' Elizabeth Ann and Mr. George Owens that used to live here. Old people they were, but they took the boy when other folks didn't want him because he limped right bad. He still is crippled some and it worries his mind that it keeps him out of the army, but other ways don't seem like it hinders him none.

"The old people that raised him didn't have no money to give him. They lived on a pension and what they could raise here on the place. But they let him go off to a school where he could work his way and get educated. And they left him this place and a horse when they died. So he ain't got no kin people.

"But Martha Lee's got too many, such as they are. She rose up out of as sorry a mess of no-count folks as the Lord ever let breathe. The whole lot of them would go to any trouble to keep out of work. It's a known fact that the daddy done enough work every year stealing from other folks to have raised a crop. But you know how now and again out of such sorry kinfolks will come a fine, honest, hard working person that makes somebody out of theyself if they get half a chance. Martha Lee is like that. Long before she was old enough, she went to work in a cotton mill. But she never had nothing for herself. It took all she made to support all that mess of kin—none of them worth killing. Then she heard about a school where she could work her way and get educated. So she just put her last pay check from the mill in her pocket and went. Her kin people disowned her for leaving home like that, and her mother told her never to darken their door again. And she ain't.

"Her and Ollie went to the same school where young people work their way. They met up with each other there, and when they got through the school they married. He's got a job in town, but they live out here because they want to raise things and because it is home to Ollie.

"I used to do for Mis' Elizabeth Ann, and my man used to work for Mr. George when they lived here. They treated us good and paid regular and give me things that was a help, specially when I took a house full of orphans to raise after my man died. So I help out these young folks and they been kind to me. When they killed hogs this fall, I helped render up the lard and make sausage, and they gave me all the chitlins and enough other meat to last up till now.

"Martha Lee wanted me to stay with her when her baby come, though she aimed to have a doctor at the birthing like you folks at the pre-mother clinic told her she needed to. Better than two weeks ago Ollie stopped by on his way to work and asked would I go stay with Martha Lee that day. She didn't feel so good. Through the day she got sicker, and when Ollie got home that evening I told him to go to the closest phone and call the doctor. You-all know they's not but two doctors in this whole county and one of them seventy-six years old and was then sick in bed with the flu. The other one had just left for the farthest end of the county with a lots of calls ahead.

"So Ollie and me had to watch over her and do the best we could. I cooked some but we didn't feel hungry and Martha Lee was in too great misery to eat. When I brought out things to cook, I saw all they had put by for winter—cured joints and side meat of two hogs, sausage and other special meat canned, uncounted jars of canned fruit and garden stuff, sorghum syrup, winter garden growing with greens and things, wood to last through the winter. A clean house and a pretty yard. Meant a lots of work and a lots of care for nice living.

"The doctor came the next night, so Martha Lee was sick two days and a night before he could get there, though he done the best he could. Ollie and his boss-man's wife phoning and sending word over the country trying to catch up with the doctor got Martha Lee's kin people informed that she was bad sick. And before the doctor came they started to get here. They caught busses and bummed rides from where they live in the edge of the next county. Her mother come, her sisters with a pack of children, menfolks—I don't know who all.

"The women folks crowded in the room with the sick girl, stood over her bed and talked loud about her dying and all the folks they knowed that died in child-bed and how it was a judgment sent on Martha Lee for leaving her kin people to starve without her wages. The men folks stomped in and out of the kitchen tracking in mud.

"When the doctor came, he cussed them all out of the room with the sick girl. They muttered around in the other room for a while and then took off their shoes and rolled into Martha Lee's nice clean beds. That got shut of them till morning and put them out of the way when the baby got borned.

"It was a pre-born baby. But you know, nurse, for you brought the incubator to warm it and keep it in.

Martha Lee's mama butted in and said she didn't want her grandbaby put in a box that looked like a coffin. And you told her if she was looking for a funeral she'd have to go somewhere else, for Martha Lee and her baby aimed to live. Then you and the doctor took Martha Lee to the hospital in the next county, us not having none.

"When Ollie went along with you-all, he asked me to shut up the house and look after things. But he didn't reckon with Martha Lee's kin people. After Ollie left they ran me off the place. Said they wouldn't leave Martha Lee's things to no old Negro woman that would tote off half the stuff on the place. Said I was so ugly I got the Bad Eye and would hoodoo folks. Said all kinds of mean things like that. When I was leaving, the daddy said he wanted some cooking before he left. 'I'm hungry enough to eat a horse and jump at the rider,' he said.

"That made me think of Ollie's horse and cow in the pasture. So I went home the back way and took them home through the fields with me to tend them. I knowed Ollie would pay me back the corn and fodder they'd eat at my place.

"A few days after that I was going to see Aunt Rosella in her trouble, and I stopped by to feed Martha Lee's chickens. Her mother came to the door and I could see other folks back in the rooms, though they were supposed to all be gone home. She said they stayed to look after things and she cussed me black and blue and slammed the door in my face. That kind of folks has one thing to hold over me that I ain't got no answer for. They're white folks—and I ain't. I thought the worst but I never let no evil thoughts run out on my tongue.

"I never come here no more till yesterday morning Ollie sent me word Martha Lee was coming and would I see if the house was clean and ready. He had been staying in town so he could catch a bus after his work and go see Martha Lee and the baby. As I came up here a buzzard flew over and cast his shadow on me—a bad sign, and I could read its meaning when I got here. Martha Lee's kin people had just left and it was a sight what this house had been through in these two weeks. Dirt—all over the place—beds filthy and tumbled up, dishes piled everywhere with greasy and sticky things dried on, floors all over red mud. Wood all burned up. Food all gone—eaten up or toted off. Two pieces of side meat, a bucket of syrup, and some canned goods all they left. The back porch all over liquor bottles and chicken feathers. I counted the chickens and made out they killed five hens. Woulda cooked more, I reckon, but it was work to pick off the feathers and riddle out the entrails.

"At the first look I thought I never could stand to clean up the mess. I couldn'ta done it but for remembering how kind the old folks and the young that lived here has been to me. Kindness is what I always wanted the best of anything and the most of. So with their kindness to give me heart, I just backed my ears and done the job. I worried my mind over the bedclothes, for seemed like I didn't have the strength to wash them. Then Ollie's boss-man's wife came out with some flowers and some baked things. And she said her washwoman could put the bed things through her electric washer. And she did and here they are all clean when Martha Lee comes home. Now in the morning I want to bring a pair of my guinea fowls for a cradle gift to the baby. Could you tell me what they named it?"

"Lee Ann," we told her, "for Martha Lee and Mis' Elizabeth Ann—for you too, Martha Lee says."

"A little white baby with my name," whispered Aunt Lee Ann, "a kindness I never dreamed of, a kindness I never dreamed of in this world."

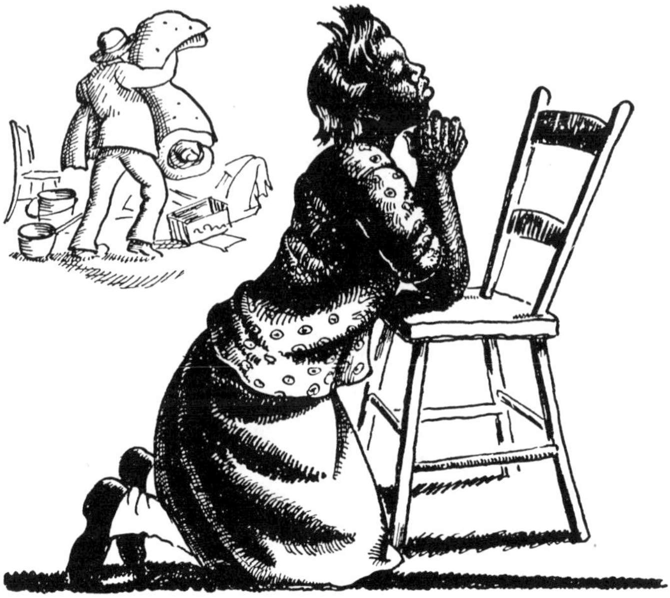

Hide and Seek with Hattie Pearl

WAY out in the country beyond the limits of her home town we overook Aunt Gussie and offered her a ride. As she settled herself on the back seat, she answered our question, "What am I doing out here in the country?" she repeated. "I'm playing hide and seek with Hattie Pearl. That's what I'm doing. Hattie Pearl had a baby two days ago—that makes fourteen—and I'm going out there to see about her and it. I just hope they still live in the same house they did two days ago. You never can tell. They move about so much. I've waited on Hattie Pearl with five babies and every time it's hide and seek to find out where they moved to last.

"People don't like for Hattie Pearl to live close to them. She's got so many children—three daughters married, married young, they did—and one dead, and this new one makes ten at home. Hattie Pearl don't try to give them any raising. She dresses up and gads about and leaves them to raise each other. They are wild and destructious. They take apart a place where they live just like a wrecking crew, and they torment the neighbors, and folks soon sends in complaints to make Hattie Pearl move. They don't pay their rent either, so they move a lots to beat the rent.

"Speaking of paying the rent, did I ever tell you, Nurse, about being at Hattie Pearl's that time the setting-out man came? Well, that was back in the days when times were so hard and jobs hard to find and the welfare people had to do so much for poor folks. But Hattie Pearl's folks don't bend their backs with work no time, good times nor bad. And they always been a trial to the welfare people.

"This day I had been over in that neighborhood to tend a sick baby all night. I was plumb tuckered out and I sat down on Hattie Pearl's porch—what there was left of it—to rest a minute. Hattie Pearl came out and asked me into the house. Her and Big Lula had been out along the railroad tracks picking wild greens and now they were sitting in the front room of Hattie Pearl's house.

"It was cluttered up and dirty with junky stuff. Three shaky old beds and a broken down cot didn't hardly leave room to walk. Hattie Pearl was sitting on the only chair in her house and it never had no back. There were plenty of boxes to sit on, though. A rusty old stove had something cooking on it and a water bucket sitting beside it. A door led off to the kitchen—for the house had two rooms.

"Hattie Pearl was making like she was reading the Bible to Big Lula. Three little children not big enough to go to school stayed out in the yard out of reach of the switch Hattie Pearl had laid across her lap. But she could reach Bethola, her foolish fitified girl that stood and stirred continuous and all the time what was cooking in the pot on the stove. And she could reach Bunch, the boy that was sitting in the front door blowing his French harp. He ought by rights to been at school, but there he sat, wearing not one thing but a suit of long underwear and a pair of shoes. He was looking down the street, and when he turned his eyes some other way, Hattie Pearl hit him with her switch. She done the same to Bethola when she stopped stirring the mess cooking in the pot.

"When I stepped in, Hattie Pearl shut up the Bible and said to Big Lula, 'I'm proud to read to my neighbor friends such gospel as I know by heart so's I can read it good. It gives me a lot of comfort knowing the Lord will provide.' Big Lula just said, 'Ain't it the truth?'

"Then Hattie Pearl said, 'He done a better job providing since the government helped the welfare people make charity more plentiful. That 'minds me, Bunch, you better watch for the Welfare Lady same time you watch for the setting-out man. I wants to tell her to give me some good clothes so I won't be shamed to show myself amongst folks dressed up for Saturday night. You hear me, Bunch?' And she hit him with the switch. He just nodded his head and went on blowing his French harp.

" 'What you get out of the Welfare Lady these days, Hattie Pearl?' Big Lula asked.

" 'Not hardly nothing we can swap for what we want worser,' Hattie Pearl told her. 'Quit'—that's her man—'did manage to dicker them two blankets for enough money to get us all in the show. But Quit said he never saw the show to do no good for watching so's the Welfare Lady wouldn't catch us using money what she calls foolish.' And she hit Bethola to make her stir faster.

"Then Bunch said real unconcerned, 'I reckon I sees the setting-out man coming a long way off!' He kept right on blowing his harp. Big Lula and Hattie Pearl went to the door to look but took care to stay hid.

"Big Lula said, 'I reckon he done caught you this time and shore going to set your things right out in the yard. The Lord have mercy!'

"But Hattie Pearl she declared, 'I ain't never been home to no setting-out man when I sees him that far off. I hides myself in the big rain barrel at the back door, being little like I am. You, Bunch, lay the lid on when I get in good.' Her and Bunch went out the back door. He came back in a minute, all the time blowing his harp. Big Lula took a dipper of water out of the bucket by the stove and threw it in Bethola's face and she fell over like in a fit. Big Lula started working with her.

"Then the setting-out man stepped in. 'How do, Mister,' said Big Lula to him.

" 'Where's Hattie Pearl?' he said without being polite about 'How do's.' 'Ain't she never home no time of day? The Law sent me to set her out of this house for not paying no rent for going on six months.'

"Big Lula kept right on working with Bethola. 'I ain't seen that Hattie Pearl,' she lied to him. 'She ain't never to her own house. Bethola took with a fit. That's how come me and Aunt Gussie here. Ain't it so, Aunt Gussie?' But I never said nothing. I ain't never been no liar and I ain't starting to lie for Hattie Pearl.

"The setting-out man looked behind the doors and under the beds. Then he went in the kitchen to make sure Hattie Pearl wasn't hid in there. Big Lula tried to turn his attention somewhere else. 'Reckon you better get us a doctor, Mister?' she asked him. 'Bethola shore been a long time in this fit.'

"He just kept right on looking. 'She'll get over her fit without no doctor,' he said. 'I reckon Hattie Pearl's off gadding like you said.'

" 'We never see her, for a fact,' Big Lula lied some more.

" 'Looks like this crew ain't going to get set out,' he

said like he was tired. 'Three months back I started serving first papers. Many's the time I had orders from the Law to set them out. But I ain't never found nobody home but a swarm of babies and that fitified girl.'

" 'Looks like you have to give it up for a bad job, Mister,' Big Lula discouraged him.

"Then seemed like he quit trying. 'I reckon I give it up for good this time,' he said. 'Ain't nobody else would live in this house noway. I hope that girl gets over her fit.' And he went out the door and started down the street. And all this time Bunch sat in the front door blowing his French harp.

"Now Bethola got up and began to stir again. Hattie Pearl came in through the kitchen door. Her and Big Lula watched the setting-out man go down the street and they laughed and hugged each other to see how he was beat out.

" 'You hear him say he done give up?' Hattie Pearl asked Big Lula. 'He shore say he quit and it sound to me like he was plumb beat out.'

"Then Bunch spoke up to say, 'The Welfare Lady coming down the street a ways. I carry her in this house to give me some pants.'

"Big Lula left, for she wanted to be at her own house when the Welfare Lady come by. But I stayed on. Bunch came in the front door with the Welfare Lady and Hattie Pearl grabbed a stumpy broom and started to sweep her house. 'How you, Miss?' she said to the Welfare Lady. 'You shore caught me before I got my house cleaned up. Bunch, drag up a place for her to sit on. Sit down, honey, for I got such trouble you can't stand to hear it lessen you sit down.'

"But the Welfare Lady just kept on standing up and Bunch blowing his harp in her ear all the while. 'Now, Hattie Pearl,' she said, 'I was here two days ago and you told me your troubles. I don't have time to listen to you today. I just stopped in to remind you again to clean up that rubbish in your yard.'

"Hattie Pearl took after Bunch and Bethola with her broom and chased them out in the yard. 'You, Bunch, and you, Bethola, get outa here and pick up that trash.' Then to the Welfare Lady, 'I layed off to do that, Miss, but not lessen there was some use going to the trouble. We been figuring to move anyhow.'

" 'Move?' said the Welfare Lady. 'I thought you were nicely settled and Quit working enough to pay the rent.'

" 'Shore, Miss, it was fixed like you say, but Quit ain't stout and he needs something to give him strength if he's got to get out and work a little. So's to save his health he let the rent slip and got a dram of liquor when he feels weak. About three months back we started getting little papers talking about setting our stuff out in the yard. Me and Quit shore has had a time dodging the setting-out man.'

" 'But, Hattie Pearl, you told me—' the Welfare Lady started to say.

" 'No, Miss,' Hattie Pearl broke in, 'I never told you nothing about this here trouble. I aimed to tote it my ownself. Me and Quit figured not to let the setting-out man find nobody at home but the least babies and

Bethola that has fits. He wouldn't never set them outdoors. It worked and now he done give up trying. I tell my younguns if he try setting things out of the house for them to keep toting things back in till he give up and quit. But he done give up and quit before it come to that.'

"The Welfare Lady done heard enough. 'Tell Quit to come see me at the office this afternoon about paying his rent. I must go now,' she told Hattie Pearl.

" 'But, Miss,' Hattie Pearl begged. 'I ain't told you nothing to give me this time. We ain't got no mattress in the house. Quit done swapped them off last week. And I ain't got no decent clothes and Bethola ain't got no shoes and Bunch ain't got no pants and—'

"The Welfare Lady just said, 'Goodbye, Hattie Pearl,' and left.

"Bethola and Bunch sneaked in the back door. Bethola started to stir in the pot again and Bunch never had quit playing his harp. 'I reckon we got to clean up this place a lots to get back on the good side of the Welfare Lady,' Hattie Pearl told them. 'You, Bunch, get outa here and pack up water to wash and scrub, if you want the Welfare Lady to give you some pants.'

" 'Who going to watch for the setting-out man?' Bunch asked his Mama. 'That my job.'

" 'He done leave us be,' said Hattie Pearl. 'Don't nobody have to watch for the setting-out man no more.'

"Right that minute the setting-out man looked in at the front door and said to Hattie Pearl, 'I reckon you won't have to watch for me after this.' And he came on in the room. For once Bunch stopped blowing his harp, but just for a minute.

"Hattie Pearl acted like the setting-out man had dropped in for a polite visit. 'How do, Mister,' she bowed to him. 'Quit ain't home. He's done been out since before good daylight scrapping up your rent money for you. He aims to carry it right down to the office you sits in.'

" 'I don't want no rent,' said the setting-out man, like he had made up his mind solid about it. 'The Law give me orders to set your stuff out in the yard, and this time I aim to do it.' Then he started gathering up covers from the beds.

"That made Hattie Pearl try a different turn. 'Now listen here, Mister,' she pleaded with him. 'You think it the Lord's will you setting folks out like you doing? Sweet Jesus never done nothing like that to poor colored folks. You need to soften your heart, Mister, you shore does. Just you lay them things down and I'll pray you the prettiest prayer you ever laid ear to.' She kneeled herself down by the chair. 'Look now,' she said, 'how I'm all ready to start soon as you lay them things down and leave us be.'

"The setting-out man just went right on to the yard with his armful of bedclothes. Hattie Pearl straightened up for a minute. 'You, Bunch, and you, Bethola, tote them things back like I told you to.' They grabbed the stuff that was piled in the yard—much of it as they could tote—and back into the house. Hattie Pearl put her head down and prayed to the rafters. The setting-out man and Bunch and Bethola kept toting things—him out, them back in. But the pile in the yard kept getting bigger and bigger faster than they could tote it back.

"Bunch poked Hattie Pearl that was still prayin loud as a trumpet, and he said to her, 'He's done got us beat out. We can't tote back fast enough.'

"Hattie Pearl straightened up and took things in the way they were. 'It shore looks like we getting set out faster'n you two younguns can set us back,' she owned up. 'I wish them teachers had kept their mouths shut about sending them other younguns to school. If they had been here to help tote, we would beat the setting-out man, shore.'

"Bunch and Bethola started to cry, but Hattie Pearl hushed them up. 'Now you-all hush up,' she gave orders. 'We ain't plumb beat out. We still got the Welfare Lady. She done told your pa to come see her about the rent. You, Bunch, go hunt somebody's pants outa that stuff in the yard and put them on.'

"The setting-out man kept right on with his work. Hattie Pearl took a little comb and looking glass out of her dress pocket and fixed herself up to go to town. She pinned Bethola's clothes together in a few places, and told the baby children huddled around me to come go with her. Bunch came in from the yard with big raggedy pants on. And they were all ready to start.

" 'You, Bunch, come to the Welfare Lady's office with our other younguns when they get out of school. Me and Bethola will get your pa from out the Greasy Spoon. Then we all go and sit in the Welfare Lady's office till she finds us a house to move in. We ain't no other way to turn. Bethola, you carry Timmy and I'll manage these two others, lessen Aunt Gussie will go along and help carry these baby children.' Hattie Pearl always draws people into her notice when she wants them to give her help. And so we left, the women folks each toting or leading a little child to town and Bunch blowing on his everlasting harp. The last time I looked back, the setting-out man had come out in the yard with the pot of stew and was standing there foolish, holding it up and not knowing what to do. Hattie Pearl she never looked back."

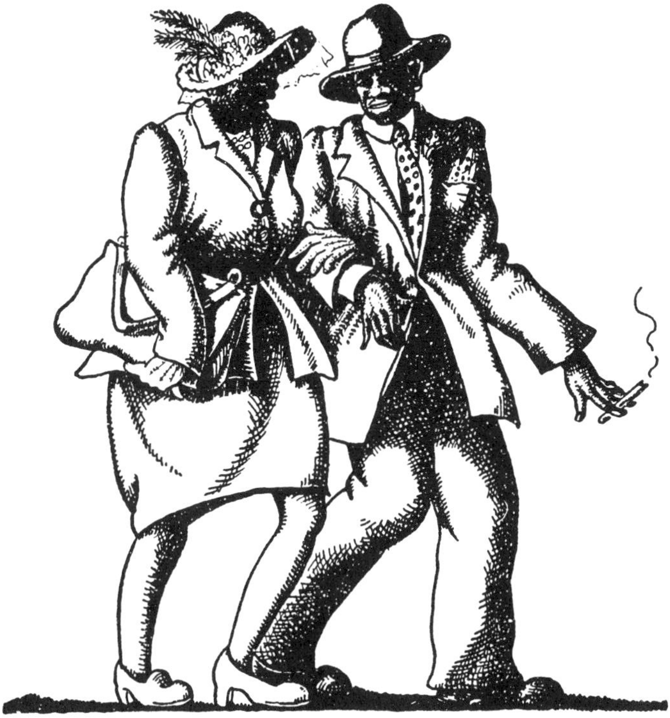

Charlie Kate and King Solomon

CHARLIE KATE has kept begging to be written about, for the main and simple reason that her husband is what she calls a "readable man" and she thinks he might "see me in printed words and find his way back to me and his own. And I wouldn't take up much room in a book. What to say about me? Go and ask Aunt Roxy. She's always knowed me from when she helped my mother birth me up to now. And she's got a gift for words which I ain't got."

Aunt Roxy was all for writing about Charlie Kate. "It wouldn't do no harm to put in a piece for her," she said. "The book folks could always throw it out if it didn't suit. And it would give Charlie Kate such pleasure, though she couldn't read it. She's everly been a person that gave out in life more than has been give back to her.

"Charlie Kate was born when her mother was middle way between forty and fifty, and her daddy was an old man. Becky, Charlie Kate's mother, hadn't had no baby for eighteen years and it was an ill-convenience to her to have one on the edge of old age. All her other children that didn't die when they was babies—and most of them did die—had gone off to Detroit and other places up North after the other big war across the ocean. That left just Becky and Joe here where they raised their family. Joe was old and disabled to work, though he had been a good worker before he broke down. They were tolerable poor and Becky had to earn all their living. Joe just pottered about the yard and wove bottoms in chairs for people, and a few odd jobs like that.

"So Becky never had time to take care of Charlie Kate good and be loving and affectionate like a baby needs. The family she worked for took up all her time. She had to go early in the morning because this white lady couldn't get her children off to school without Becky. They had young girls in the family and done a lot of entertaining, so they kept Becky late at night a lot of times. When Charlie Kate was a baby, about the only time Becky saw her awake was on Sundays when she got off from work after noon dinner. Then she dressed up the baby and took her to church. That has made Charlie Kate always a big worker in the church.

"The white lady she worked for didn't try to give Becky no extra time for the baby, because she was mad at Becky for having a baby, a big piece of foolishness she called it at Becky's time of life. She never hardly gave Becky time to have the baby, because one of her girls was having a wedding and they couldn't manage the wedding without Becky.

"So there was only the old man to look after little Charlie Kate. He made such a mess of trying to fix her bottles to feed her that one of my girls that had a new baby nursed Charlie Kate too till she could eat cooked things. Neighbors helped out old Joe and sometimes the roomers did a turn for the baby.

"Becky and Joe owned a house in the good part of the colored end of town—close to the fire station. They had five rooms but rented out three of them to splice out Becky's wages to live on.

"Charlie Kate never had much chance to play and be with other children. Her daddy got older and more helpless and she had to stay close at home and watch after him, even when she was a little bitty thing. Other children wouldn't come there to play in her yard because they were afraid of Joe—Devil Joe they called him. He wasn't mean, though, just looked queer and acted strange and that made folks scared of him. All the time he got more queer and his mind got bad. Charlie Kate couldn't go to school, for watching her daddy so close all the time. About the most pleasure she got was to potter among the flowers in the yard with him and once in a long while take little trips with him to the woods to dig up things to plant. She learned from him to weave chair bottoms and did that work when he got past knowing how.

"His mind got worse, and one day he raked leaves and sticks under the house and, like an unknowing child, was fixing to set fire to it. Charlie Kate couldn't make him stop. So she ran to the fire station and when the fire engine got to the house, Joe had already fired the leaves and trash under the house. They put out the blaze with little damage. But after that Becky had to put Joe away with crazy folks, where he didn't live long. Charlie Kate was then thirteen years old and big for her age and too proud to start to school that late in life and have to sit with the babies.

"So Becky started taking Charlie Kate with her to work to help her and so's not to leave Charlie Kate by herself. Becky was getting old, and before long Charlie Kate was doing most of her work. Becky went along every day to guide and show Charlie Kate, and see that the young man in the family kept himself to himself. He might get smart with a young girl like Charlie Kate alone but not with Becky there. She helped raise him and he knowed to mind her better than he minded his white mama.

"Then Becky died when Charlie Kate was seventeen, and some of their folks up North came back home for the funeral. They got mad, though, because Becky had willed Charlie Kate the house. So they treated Charlie Kate right bad and never so much as said, 'Will you come home with us for a visit to lighten your burden of sorrow?'

"Charlie Kate kept her mother's old work place. The children in the family was all married and gone off, except to come back on a visit. So the work was lighter for Charlie Kate. I went up to her house to live with her, for company and for protection. And I lived there till Charlie Kate married and now I live there again.

"She had friends among the men folks before, but none of them seemed to reach her affections and none of them was the fast-marrying kind till King Solomon Simms came up from Florida. Charlie Kate met him at a church social. He was all dressed up like a lawyer and his talk was full of educated words and he had such loving ways. The loving ways touched Charlie Kate deep, for she had always been hungry for loving affection.

"So she was right ready to say yes when he asked her would she marry him. Like I said, Charlie Kate was always good to work in the church. On her next day off from work after she promised to marry King Solomon, she went with the ladies from her church to make war bandages at the Red Cross. There was a white lady there from the college to oversee the colored church workers. She had on a red tailor-made suit that struck Charlie Kate's fancy.

"After the work stopped, Charlie Kate asked the white lady how did she think a red suit like that would do for a wedding dress. The lady said she was partial to white or blue to get married in, but maybe a red dress would suit Charlie Kate better. Then Charlie Kate asked where could she get a dress like that. And the lady said if Charlie Kate would do her ironing and pack her suit satchel for a trip the next week, she would make Charlie Kate a dress like hers for the wedding. So it was a bargain.

"The lady bought the goods in Atlanta, and on Charlie Kate's next day off she made a red suit and a yellow blouse like Charlie Kate wanted instead of a white blouse like hers. Charlie Kate got a yellow hat and yellow gloves to match. And her outfit made a pretty picture, though the red suit fit her more spread out than the white lady's because Charlie Kate was some eighty pounds bigger than her. King Solomon Simms came and waited to walk home with Charlie Kate from the college lady's home and was as polite as a basket of chips.

"The wedding was in the church. Her sisters in the church dressed the house for the wedding with japonicas, and January jessamine and kiss-me-at-the-gate, things that bloom right soon after Christmas. The college lady and some of Charlie Kate's other white folks came to the wedding and brought her presents. The next night Charlie Kate had a part in the church play. She wore her wedding outfit and never looked so pretty nor so happy before. She was eating her white bread then.

"They had a nice honeymoon. The folks Charlie Kate worked for took her to New York with them to take care of their grandbaby on the way there and back. They bought her a fine black dress and some fancy white aprons and caps to wear. And she had a nice trip on the sleeping cars. The colored people who worked for the family her white folks were visiting treated her good and took her places to see the big city. Charlie Kate's husband went to Memphis with a friend that was driving a transport truck. Charlie Kate gave her husband some of her money to spend on the trip when he said he was a little short of cash after the wedding. Her trip and everything connected was all furnished to her. Going different places that way, they had more to tell each other when they got back than if they went to the same place. I never did hear what he did in Memphis, but Charlie Kate told over and over to ready ears about her trip to New York.

"After that trip Charlie Kate settled down to work again. Her husband said he would hate to take her away from her white folks. And anyhow, he said, he hadn't found just the kind of work yet that suited his talents to do. Then he talked to Charlie Kate about having her house made over in his name. He said that was according to the law so it would fall to him if anything happened to her. Charlie Kate told me about it and I told her she better go up to Mr. Bob's law office and take two dollars and tell him she wanted that much worth of advice in the law. She done that and he said, "You can't make over your house to nobody, for it's not all yours by yourself. Your folks up North got a claim on it." That weren't the pure truth, for Becky willed the house to just Charlie Kate and nobody else. But Mr. Bob had to satisfy her that she *couldn't* make her house over to King Solomon or she would have done it; she was so wrapped up in loving that man.

"After that, he left Charlie Kate and she grieved herself nearly about sick. Every day after work she went by the college lady's house and had her write long loving letters to King Solomon begging him to come back. After a month or so he came back from where he had been living out in the country with another girl and Charlie Kate was too happy to see straight. Then he left again and was clear gone.

"I talked Charlie Kate into going to the pre-mother clinic the health nurses and doctor had. They found out she had caught bad blood from King Solomon and needed to take shots to make her well and her baby live and be healthy. When she told the folks she worked for that she had to get off regular every Monday to take shots for bad blood, they wanted to fire her for fear they would catch it from her. But the health nurse talked to them and said Charlie Kate would be safe enough if she took her shots regular. So they were glad to keep her.

"About two months before she got down, Charlie

Kate had to quit work because she wasn't able to go no longer. Then she had just her rent money to live on. So she rented the part of her house she lived in and took a bed and a few things to live in an old one room shack that had been a store in the worst part of Dogtown. That was where she lived when she sent for me. I found her there by herself on a dark chilly night in the fall. No light but an old lamp with no chimney and no oil. No wood and nothing to make wood. I lit my big lantern that I always tote along with me on night cases. Charlie Kate had been there down sick in the bed two days and nobody to do for her.

"I remembered a good pile of wood at her preacher's house. So I woke him up out of bed, and he filled the back of his car with wood and took it to Charlie Kate. I got old Aunt Mattie to stay with me through the night. She couldn't do nothing but sit and be company for me. So the night passed.

"Charlie Kate's baby was twins, nice little girls. She named them Georgia and Florida for hers and her husband's home states. That man, wherever he was, got word about the twins and came back to Charlie Kate. He said he never had occasioned the birth of twins before and he was mighty proud. Charlie Kate was so happy to see him she got up out of the bed and cooked him a fine dinner out of stuff he brought in. She made good crusty corn pone, fried catfish, cooked greens with a ham bone, and made fried apple pies. She got as hot as a depot stove, and the babies were just four days old. So she was bad sick for a while after that.

The neighbors came and waited on her and her white folks brought her things. Her husband stayed around, but he never so much as toted in a turn of wood.

"He did bring in the money and they lived good for a few weeks. It was cotton harvest time and he made a pile of money gambling with colored men that had their cotton money in their pockets. Then one night sudden he took a notion to go to New York where he said he could get the kind of jobs he ought to have and rights of a citizen like a white man. That sounded mighty fine to Charlie Kate, remembering her honeymoon trip to New York. And she would have followed her King Solomon to the jumping off place anyhow. The right reason he wanted to go to New York quick was that him and another colored man had shot at each other over a gourd of water and a woman—but that's another story, not for me to tell right now. He was just a low-flung coward running off from the Law. But he didn't tell Charlie Kate any of that. He told her lies plain and fancy, and she believed him right down to the ground. They left in the night and Charlie Kate gave me her keys and told me to collect her rents for her.

"This trip to New York weren't no honeymoon. It's a mercy Charlie Kate lived to tell about that trip on buses with two young babies. And she had no friends there where she went this time. One room in a kind of cellar in the big colored part of town where he took her to live. Pitch dark in her room in broad day without the light turned on. No yard, no sun, all smells.

Folks above on all sides grumbled and growled when the babies cried. And her husband leaving her there all day and into the night by herself, scared to death and sick with the strange, crowded, lonesome feeling she had. Then one day he got on a screeching black train that went tearing away under the ground into the dark and he never came back to Charlie Kate any more. Day in and day out she waited, but no King Solomon. Then some welfare people helped her to get back down home here with her babies. And she went back to her old job.

"The Lord viewed me to retire from being a granny-midwife and step down off the Board and help Charlie Kate take care of her twin babies. So we live together in her two rooms of her house. And I've got my little pension money to live by myself again if King Solomon ever comes back to her. And day and night she longs for him to come back. One time I said to her, 'How can you love a man that acts so miserable mean in this world? Whatever did he give you?'

"And she said, 'He ain't ever give me nothing but Georgia and Florida. But how I do love him is untelling.' "

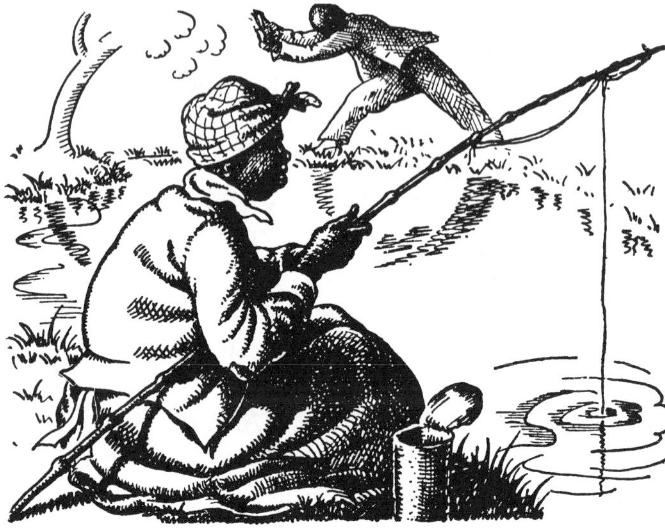

An Ill-Convenience

OVER and over the granny-midwives ask one another and their nurses, "How can you make them notice you ahead of time?" It is not being dragged out in the middle of the night that they complain of, but being "jerked up at the last minute" by patients whom they are not expecting to care for. "It is such an ill-convenience not to have notice beforehand," they say.

Aunt Kansas complains, "Just let me think about going fishing. No, they don't stop me before I get started. They wait till I takes a dozen and three eggs to the store and says, 'Give me that much fish hooks,' then till I've dug me some worms and got settled on the creek bank with fish starting to nibble on my bait. Then there comes tearing across the fields some urgent man hollering that his wife needs me quick. Maybe I have to set there with her the whole day, but anyhow I'm done fishing."

Another complains that she can never wash her quilts or make a kettle of soap without being called to a birthing. Still another says she couldn't eat her Christmas dinner in peace this year for having to leave in the middle of it. Tales of missing the sermon at church are numerous.

Finally comes Aunt Kansas' story of going to the plays at the church. "It was two-three years before the war," she said. "And the colored folks were having some plays at the church. Not having cash to speak of except cotton picking time and none to brag about then, living on furnished rations and credit, us colored folks always knowed how to have fun without money to spend, though the war has changed that a lots even way out in the country where I lives. So one way we had fun was to act out plays. Sometimes a few white folks come to see our plays, but mostly they paid no mind to our sociable doings amongst ourselves.

"One of these here plays was a homemade play and the other one came out of the Bible. Hannah and the school teacher trained the people to speak their words and act out their manners. And when the time came, I said to myself, 'Maybe I can go in peace. No babies as I knows of near at hand. So I went early and got me a front seat. And I prayed to the Lord not to let nobody come tipping down the aisle and whisper to me to come in a hurry. And I reckon He heard me.

"The homemade play came first. It was called 'What Will a Man Choose?' After a big commotion behind the sheets that made curtains for the stage, the curtains parted wide and the announcer came out and explained what it was all about. But folks were still coming in late and so we couldn't hear what he said. So we had to just catch the idea as best we could.

"First some little children came out dancing. That meant teeniny children didn't have to get fogged up with choosing or pressed down with not having no choice. They didn't have no set steps but had instructions to dance like they felt happy. They all had on little thin white shimmies of tobacco cloth cut off at their knees to save goods. The church had new electric lights from the power line across the country and they had fixed lights to shine underfoot at the front of the stage. When they turned the lights on, it looked like it melted away them little white shimmies to a thin mist, and the little black bodies shone through same as if the little children were naked. They didn't know, and danced sweet and pretty and lively too, while Jake played tunes on his French harp.

"Then the things for folks to choose in life began to come out when the announcer told about them. There were two kinds of folks to show Good Times. One was a girl wearing a blue satin dress with a bustle in the back that she acted more with than any other part.

She had high-heel shoes, and a fancy hairdo and had her hands full of hot dogs and coca colas. Then there were folks with a banjo and a coon dog and a fishing pole and a watermelon and things like that to have good times with.

"The man that played Money was dressed on top of his clothes, front and back, with big dollar bills tall as he was, painted on store wrapping paper to look like natural money. He just came out and sat for a minute on a cotton bale and then went off out of sight.

"Lige Hampton from the filling station was called Service. He wore his filling station clothes and acted like he was waiting on a car and wiping the glass, and all that.

"One of the preachers was called Religion. And he showed off with preaching a sermon on a knothole. Just to prove you can talk in a moralizing way about anything at all, he said. But I don't see no use to stretch your moralizing that far to cover a knothole.

"Politics was fixed with a false face to look like a white man, the only one in the play he was. But let me pass over a lot of folks fixed up to be something or other in life. Let me pass over to tell you the best part.

"That was the last part and it was called Hard Work. It was so natural to life you felt like you were up there acting it out yourself. First came the Plowing, just men—not with mules nor plows—but they made out their parts with actions and songs till you could fairly see the pokey old mules and smell fresh dirt as it turned up a new furrow. Then came the Cotton

Chopping and Cotton Picking with all the family in the cotton patch down to the least babies on pallets in shady places or in cotton baskets. They worked and they sang so natural to life the rest of us joined in in spite of ourselves. And so that homemade play ended up with everybody in the whole church house acting a part. Though that weren't in the plans, it couldn't end no other way.

"The next play was from the Bible and called 'Mordecai's Housetop.' You-all know that story about the Jew girl named Esther that had married the King because she was so pretty and because her uncle was clever in politics. Her uncle's name was Mordecai and he was a Jew. A lot of folks in that country hated Jews. Maybe it was Germany. Anyhow I don't know the name of the country. There was a big politician named Haman that hated Jews like poison. He figured how could he get rid of them, and he thought of hanging and fixed a hanging place ready. Then he went around with a little book taking down the names of all the Jews to get them sorted out from the other folks that lived there. In the play, there he was writing and writing in his little old book of doom till he nearly 'bout had all the Jews' names put down. And there was Mordecai finagling around in politics, not knowing he would be the first Jew Haman would hang, not knowing about Haman's plot against all the Jews.

"Then the word came on the grapevine to Esther that all her kin people, the Jews, would get killed if she didn't make the King do something quick. Seemed like they had been married a mighty long time, for it had got to where she had to wait to be sent for to keep company with the King. If she went when he didn't want her to, he might get mad enough to chop off her head. She knowed all that but she didn't hang back afraid. She just got up her spunk, and dressed herself pretty, and went to the room where the King sat on a throne.

"The King was Jake, and Esther, the queen, was his sister Hannah. She looked every inch a queen standing there in the door with a golden crown made out of shower-of-gold flowers. She looked at the King and then she sang to him the song, 'There's a Man Going Round Taking Names.' Hannah always gets people excited when they hear her sing. Jake weren't no exception. He got excited and forgot his play speech and just said to her, 'Come in, howdy.'

"Hannah kept her queen's manners and knelt down in front of him and sang 'Let My People Go.' That melted his heart with love of his queen and with pity for her kin people. And so the Jews were saved from hanging. Then he got rid of Haman and tore up his little book full of names. After that he gave Mordecai a high office in politics that paid good money, not through no virtue of Mordecai—but that's the way of politics.

"When he had got Mordecai set up in politics, the King sent for the school teacher to come and write down all that had took place, so it would be in the history books to his credit. And the King touched the pen because he couldn't write his name. Then he made it a law for everybody to let the Jews alone to live in peace. And he sent the police to ride around over the country and say that was the law.

"With his business finished up, the King told folks to go 'long home and leave him and his queen be by theyselves. Then he said to her, 'Let's you and me sing some to celebrate what we done this day.' So him and Esther, the queen, stepped to the front and sang for us.

"Nobody joined in like in the end of the homemade play. When Jake and Hannah sing together, just them two, it lifts us up past singing ourselves. They sang on into the night—the old songs that come up to us from slavery days when black people made their songs to be a way to reach from the lowly earth up to high heaven to touch the heart of God."

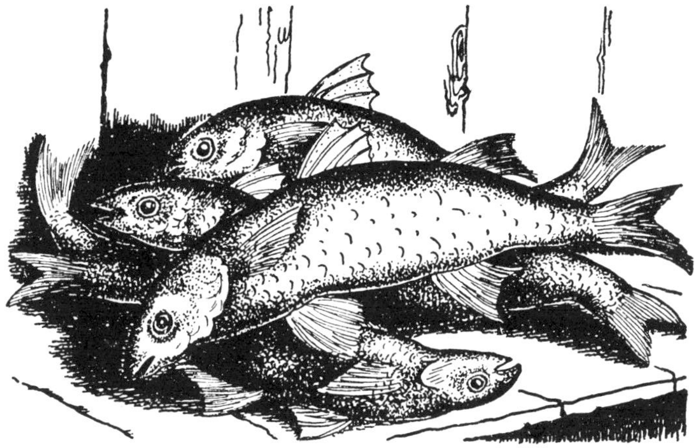

Walker's Hack Is the Safest

THE crowd had just begun to gather for a mullet supper at the colored church. The evening air was thick with the smell of frying fish and the smoke of mosquito smudges. A little group of old grannies had gathered on the steps of the church for a sociable chat in the shelter of the smudge they had set near by. After the usual inquiries about health and disinterested remarks about the weather, the talk warmed up to stories of their experiences as grannies. This time the stories centered around adventures in various kinds of transportation.

"Mostly I take walker's hack," said one old woman, telling how often she had no way of getting to a case but to walk. "But that don't make no story to tell."

So she told of clinging on behind a young Negro on a motorcycle, rushing to his wife whom she had promised to deliver. Another told of riding in an ox cart as a contrast to the reckless speed of her sister midwife on a roaring motorcycle. Aunt Lovetta told about the time a halfgrown boy came to take her to his mother and brought a mule for her to ride. "It was all well enough," she said, "till we came through town. Then that mule took it into his head to act foolish and he went charging up the wide courthouse steps to the long veranda that stretched across the front of the courthouse. He brayed loud two times and then went down the steps slow and easy. Me on his back all that time and the whole crowd of courthouse loafers and workers laughing at the Wild West Show."

"I've traveled to a baby case every way but to fly or swim," declared Aunt Doll. "And there were times when I thought I might swim. Before they put that bridge across the river, I was scared twist-legged every time I had to be set across the river in a boat, afraid I'd get spilled out in the water and have to swim or drown."

"You don't know the first thing about being scared in a boat," Aunt Doffie interrupted. "Just let me tell what happened to me when I lived on one of the Georgia sea islands. One night it was dark as black cats stacked up in a pile and the water was rough when a man came for me to tend on his wife. After I got in the boat and way out on the dark water the boat kept going every which a-way. At first I thought it was the rough water. Then it come to me in a flash that the man was ape drunk and couldn't manage that boat no more than a rabbit, even in smooth water. All my life I'd been used to travel in boats, but not in the middle of the night on bad waters with the only other person in the boat ape drunk.

"We'll pass over all the trembling and praying I done and not use up a lot of words telling how it scared the fool out of me to know the fix I was in. We'll pass over to when the boat started to go right again and head for the shore. The water was rough as ever and I looked about to see what brought the change for the better. And there guiding the boat steady and sure sat the best-looking pirate man you ever saw. He was dark skinned, though I don't think he was a man of color but maybe a Spaniard or some other kind of dark white man. He had fine gold earrings nearly down to his shoulders, good heavy pirate earrings, not no fancy little womanish earbobs. He had on pirate boots and he had jewels flashing in the handle of his dagger or some kind of cutting weapon hung on his belt. Shore, I could see what he had on. The night was black like I said, but he had a curious little old lantern that made a circle of light around him. From the time I was a little child I had heard tales of pirates that used to come around the Georgia sea islands but never I give much thought to how one would look for I never hoped to see one. But soon as I laid eyes on him I said to myself, 'That is a pirate shore as I'm born.' I was born with a veil on and so I got a good sense of ghosts and such things. That's why I knowed him so soon and why I wasn't scared of the pirate, though I was scared of that fool drunk man out on the sea in a boat.

"Well, we landed on the shore and I helped pull up the boat and tie it. We left the man laying in the boat, for I didn't need him one bit around his wife's house and him dead asleep now with rotgut liquor. I turned around to thank the pirate kindly, but he had already gone on ahead up the dark path to light me a way to the house. As I went in the door of the house, he just melted away in the outside darkness.

"I thought to myself, 'That's the last of him.' But no. When the baby was born and I wrapped it up and turned to lay it down, there was the pirate holding out his arms for the baby. Now I was in a fix. I couldn't give a live baby to a ghost even if he did have a kind look on his face. And I didn't want to make a pirate mad at me. So I just used my ghost sense and laid the baby in the chair and let the pirate stand and watch over it while I tended the mother. When I looked again for him, he was gone off.

"After that I pieced together in my mind what tales I had heard about pirates on that island. When I pieced together the scraps I had the story about a pirate, young and good-looking and rich, that used to come to this island some generations back. He fell in love with a girl on the island and she done the same with him. He made big risks for himself coming to court her and wanted to marry her. But the girl's father wouldn't hear none of it, for he thought the pirate's trade was evil and all pirates brothers of the devil. So he drove the pirate off to the wide seas.

"When the girl's baby was born, her father threw it into the sea. If it was born dead or alive I don't know. Then he took the girl far off some place where nobody never heard tell of them again. When the young pirate came back he heard about the baby and he hunted a long time for its little corpse. He hunted for the girl too. For years he came back now and then to look. Then you see when he died his ghost come back to that island. And the house I went to was on the place where his lover had lived. So naturally he could take me there in the dark.

"The next year there was another baby and it was born dead. The pirate held out his arms for it. And, being as it was dead, I told him to sit down in the chair and I laid it on his lap. He looked happy and I don't know how long he sat there. After that I used to see him at all my birthings on that island. He never come till the baby was born and he always held out his arms for it, though I never let him touch a living baby. Now and again I thought I caught glimpses of him other places, but I couldn't be sure, for he wasn't wearing his pirate earrings and other pirate things.

"About that time he started leaving presents for me. Mostly it was fish. Every morning there would be a mess of fresh fish at my door, or fresh crabs, or little pretty sea shells or things like that. Always things from out the water, a sign of the pirate. Then I glimpsed him a few times when he left presents for me at the door of my house before day.

"Pretty soon my man began to ask questions about these things left for me at my house. This man of mine had a jealous heart. You know I ain't never had no luck with my men. The first one just got restless and went off and never come back. That was when I was right young and a baby coming every year. The first man was good to me but young and restless. The next two were good men and helped me raise our children and mine but they didn't neither one live long. One got drowned out of a boat and the other one got killed on a Saturday night in town.

"This one I had when the pirate come to me was a mean-tempered man. His name tree must had rough bark, he had such a mean temper. I met up with him at the praise house and he was the best singer of the shout songs in the whole congregation. So I thought he would be a good man for me. But he didn't hold out good the week through. On week days he sang bad-man songs and lived according. He had no cause to complain about me or treat me bad, for I kept my house mother-clean and stayed with him faithful and gave him part of my wages. All the children were grown up and gone, so he never had a houseful of children to fret him.

"Naturally I couldn't tell him about no pirate that was kind to me because I tended little babies and the pirate was lonesome for his little baby he never did see. So my man took the notion some other men was running after me. And he followed me with a sharp razor when I went out on a case at night. But he never did see no man with me. My husband didn't have no ghost sense, so he never got the least glimpse of the pirate. Nights when I was at home—and mostly I was, for babies come occasional—my man took to sleeping with a big sharp sugar cane knife that looked like murder itself. Now if you ain't never went to bed with a mean-hearted man and a big bloodthirsty cane knife, you don't know what it is to sleep restless. Of course I knowed he couldn't hurt my pirate friend with no cane knife, the pirate being a ghost without blood and meat on his bones. But the cane knife shore could hack me into sausage meat.

"So I tried to drive away the pirate and his presents from the sea. I planted mustard seed under the front steps and under the gate sill. When that never drove away the ghost with fish and other things to give me, I tried salt and pepper and collard seeds in the same places. I slept with the Bible under my pillow to keep off ghosts, good or bad. Then I took out the Bible and put a sifter under the pillow for a charmer away of spirits. But every morning sure as daylight there would be the present from the pirate waiting for me.

"After a time I went to a conjure woman to get help to drive off the friendly pirate. She made up a strong conjure bag with hog bristles and black cats' hair and a rabbit's foot and dirt from the graves of seven murderers and seven little stones from south-running water all tied up in a red flannel rag greased with snake oil and tied with dead woman's hair. With faith in the conjure bag I slept easier that night, but woke up the next morning to the prettiest mess of mullet you ever saw. So I gave up trying to drive off the pirate.

"All the time my man got meaner and beat me unmerciful and whetted up his sugar cane knife every night before he went to bed. Every way I knew I tried to drive him off peaceful. I put some of his hairs in the gills of a fish and let it swim away. I tried all the charms I could find out to make him go off and leave. But every night there was him and his cane knife laying up in my bed. So I just resigned from living with him and slipped off into the back country to live away from the sea islands and the sea, where the pirate wouldn't come. Not long after that my man was killed mysterious with his own sugar cane knife and I always thought the pirate done the killing to rid me of a danger to my life.

"No, I ain't had no other man since then. I go by the name of my first man now. He had such a fine-sounding name, Littleberry Strange. And I ain't had no ride in a boat since then. I don't go on no cases I can't walk to. I done learned that walker's hack is the safest way for me to travel."

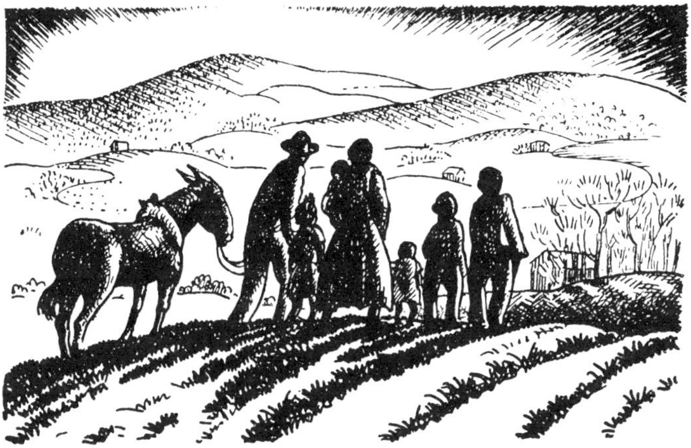

Two Suit Satchels Made of Carpet Goods

THE little black leather bags which the midwives use to carry their equipment and supplies in do wear out, and just now they are hard to replace. Midwives continually ask nurses, and nurses continually ask supply companies, "Where can we get midwife bags and when?"

Aunt Jeanie solved the problem for herself by bringing out a family heirloom, an ancient carpetbag. I saw her carrying it at a meeting where nurses inspected midwife bags and equipment; and I thought at the time, "I bet my hat that old carpetbag has a history." When later I had a chance to ask Aunt Jeanie, she brought the carpetbag out for me to look at closely and told me how her family came to have it.

"We got two suit satchels made of carpet goods in our family," Aunt Jeanie began. "One of them is a precious keepsake from a friend and we keep it put away nice and never use it. Mama gave it to my sister, Robert E. Lee—Mam Bob everybody calls her now that we are old. This one Mama gave to me and I always used it some, for we never thought so much of it as to put it by just for a keepsake. And this is how come we have these two carpet goods suit satchels in our family.

"The one Mama gave to my sister belonged to a thoroughly good white man that was a good friend to Mama and her family. He came from a place called Massachusetts with two trunks full of books and a fine violin. He came to the South to teach in a private school for young ladies. Nobody but Colonel Foster ever knew the story of why he came, and Colonel Foster never did tell. It couldn't have been a bad reason why he came, on account of he done so much good after he got here. When people got curious about it, Mama always said it would be ill-bred to ask questions. In the daytime he taught the young ladies languages and music, and he lived at Colonel Foster's big plantation house. Of nights he took another job teaching colored folks.

"At Colonel Foster's, the ladies in the family taught reading to a good many of the colored women that worked about the house and to house boys and some of the smartest children. But the men and the women field hands had no chance to learn. The schoolmaster talked about it with Colonel Foster and they agreed with each other that ignorant work hands weren't the best to have on your place, though most men with slaves believed contrary to Colonel Foster and the schoolmaster.

"Some work hands that could carpenter fixed up an old building that stood down by the edge of the big garden to have the colored people's school in. And at night the schoolmaster taught them to read and write and figure a little, if they wanted to learn. Nobody was made to learn anything if he didn't choose. Mostly these work hand scholars come from Colonel Foster's plantation, but some other white men let a few of their slaves come who wanted to read. Not many though, for most of the plantation men and town folks too were mad at Colonel Foster and said he was laying up trouble. They rode up on their fine horses to argue him out of it. Mama heard a lot of the talk, for she was head cook at the Fosters' big house.

"These men said wait and see Colonel Foster's slaves would get so smart they would rise up against him someday. And they would run off and leave him no hands to work his place. Colonel Foster just said, 'Damn it to hell, this is my business.' The folks that argued with Colonel Foster missed their guess. When the war was being fought and after freedom, more colored folks stayed on Colonel Foster's place than any other. And there was more peaceful times and more to eat amongst the Fosters and their hands in those bad times because all the Foster folks worked and raised things to eat.

So the schoolmaster's teaching never spoiled the Foster Negroes like folks prophesied it would. Besides teaching his black scholars, the master would play fine music for them on his violin or read poetry. He said to rest them from the day's work before they started to work learning things out of books. Mama said one time she heard Colonel Foster talking with the schoolmaster about the music and the poetry, after Colonel Foster had been to the colored folks' school, and Colonel Foster said, 'My God, man, it takes civilized men to do common labor all day and then wash themselves and sit and listen to great music and poetry!' And the schoolmaster said, 'That is what you saw . . .' And Mama didn't hear the rest.

"After he came back from fighting in the war with our men, the schoolmaster helped nurse the wounded soldiers that came back from the war. His school for young ladies hadn't opened up again yet. When the colored folks pulled off from the white folks' churches, he done a good thing training colored preachers to read and to speak better. . . .

"But I started to tell you about the suit satchels. To end that story, he gave Mama the keepsake suit satchel to carry his laundry in. After the war she didn't have so much work at the Fosters', for there weren't so much fine stuff to cook and no big parties for a few years. So she washed and ironed the schoolmaster's shirts and things. One day the children carrying his fresh ironed clothes dropped some in the mud and Mama had to wash them over. He felt so bad about the extra work for Mama that he gave the suit satchel to her to carry his clothes back and forth in.

"Now this suit satchel I'm using for my granny midwife things . . . One night after the war and freedom a white man came home with Papa, carrying two suit satchels—this is one of them. Papa said this man believed in equality and brotherhood of man and wanted to stay all night at our house. Mama said white folks traveling through the country stayed up at the Fosters' big house. And Papa said in the kitchen that the man said he guessed he'd get a cold welcome up there. That made Mama say that white folks too trashy to stay at the Fosters' were beneath her notice. Then Papa told Mama this man was going to help him get set up in politics and get him a mule and forty acres of ground. Mama said that wasn't nothing but a big Yankee lie, and my little sister said was this man a Yankee, and Mama said, 'Don't us use that word *Yankee* for folks from up North, for that would include the schoolmaster in, and he is heaven's wideness above this man that come home with your papa.'

"The man stayed anyhow. Mama got supper at the Fosters' and brought the children some, and she made the children sit out in the yard and eat their supper from the Fosters'. Then she fixed a snack for Papa's company and tried to make the cooking as bad as she could. Mama had to try hard to cook bad. Papa and the man went off together and came back way in the night. They lay around the next day and talked politics. That night they went off again and Papa whispered and told Mama they were going to a meeting called the Union League.

"After they left Mama put on a pair of Papa's old pants and a cap and followed them. She watched the League meeting in the woods with a big bunch of colored folks and some more white men like the one at our house, filling the air with talk of politics and big promises. Papa was the only Foster Negro there and that worried Mama. She had to get that white man out of our house or he'd ruin Papa's good name. She slipped back to our house and woke up my two little brothers and told them to do what she said, after Papa and the man came back, and they were always good to mind.

"After a while Papa and the man came in and the man got in Mama's nice front room bed where she fixed for him to sleep by himself, while the rest of us stacked up together in the other room beds. Next morning the man woke up with my two little brothers in the bed with him and one of them had branched in the bed and the man was all wet. That was what Mama told my little brother to do when they crawled in with the man after he was asleep, though Mama would have whipped my brother sore for doing such a trick any other time. The man was so mad he said bad and dirty things about nasty little niggers in the bed with him. It wouldn't do to tell. Mama said what about equality and brotherhood ideas, but he just cussed and swore and left out so mad and in a big rush that he left behind this suit satchel with two old pairs of pants and a stack of printed papers in it.

"Of course Papa was raring mad and said Mama had ruined his chances in politics. That night he went to the League meeting again. And Mama slipped off and followed him again. That night was darker and she got lost for a little coming home. So Papa got home first and caught her as she came in and found out where she had been to. He was mad and said he would tell the League on her for sneaking up and listening to their secret meetings. He just meant to scare Mama because he was so mad at her.

"But when he told the League on Mama, he stirred up trouble. The suit satchel man that stayed at our house was the ringleader, and he was crazy mad at Mama. So he stirred up the Leaguers against her, saying she would let out their secrets and she was in a plot with the white folks to keep them from their rights as citizens and all such lies as that. The upshot of it was the League court-martialed Mama and sentenced her to hang the next morning there in the woods where she spied on their meetings—all the proceedings to be a dead secret. They didn't think Papa would let out the secret, for he was the one told on Mama in the first place.

"Papa sure was one scared man. He never did want Mama hanged or harmed no way. He just wanted her scared when he was mad at her for meddling in his business. There wasn't but one thing for Papa to do and that was to tell the Fosters. When he told them, they got busy in a hurry and sent Papa to bring the sheriff while Colonel Foster and the schoolmaster and others in the family—even two of the young ladies—rode out to get men from all over the country. While they were gone some of the League members slipped in the back way and stole Mama and left the children screaming in a fright.

"The sheriff and two deputies rode to where Papa told them the League met and they told the Leaguers to turn Mama a-loose. They wouldn't do it and talked smart against the Law. So the sheriff and his deputies rode back to meet with the other men gathering in from over the country. The Leaguers were fixing a rope to hang Mama to save their secrets, and they were bragging how they scared off the sheriff, when a big troop of horses come breaking through the underbrush. And there was circled around two sides of them—men from all over the country—white men and boys and a lot of colored folks too. Come to save Mama. Some of them on horses and more a-foot—with guns and war swords. Not no Ku-Klux, not no masks and robes, just folks in their everyday clothes come to help a colored woman out of trouble. The Leaguers dropped their rope in a hurry and scattered wide and fast through the swamps where they fell behind logs and lay there too scared to breathe. Nobody followed them up or killed any of them, for the whole point was to save Mama; Mandy was the name all folks knew her by. They brought Mama home and Colonel Foster said to Papa, 'Rome, we brought Mandy back to you safe. Take good care of her or you'll have the devil to pay.'

"The suit satchel man never did come back. Mama

gave the children his papers to play with and made the two little brothers pants out of the pants he left behind in the suit satchel. Papa never did rise up in politics. He voted as long as colored people had the vote—good many years it was. But he never did let no white man with a carpet goods suit satchel tell him who to vote for. I think Mama always told him, though she never would own up to it.

"No, Papa never rose in politics but he was a leader amongst the colored people and done a heap of good in his time. He was a good worker and had such an honest name any man would trust him with anything he owned or give him credit without signing papers. All our family always had as good a name as Papa way back beyond and up to now, all except St. Paul, and I reckon any good family has one rascal in it about every third generation.

"There came a time when Papa owned thirty acres of land and a mule of his own. Mama sent for the married children to come home and visit and see when he got the deeds. And he showed us the deeds and the mule and he said to us, 'We got land now and live property!' And we all walked together all over our thirty acres and led our mule behind us to see and to feel the land under our feet. And Papa kept saying to us, 'We got land now and live property,' and Mama laughed at him and said, 'Yes, Rome, we got good land and we earned it with our own hard work. It shore didn't come by politics nor out of no carpet goods suit satchel.' "

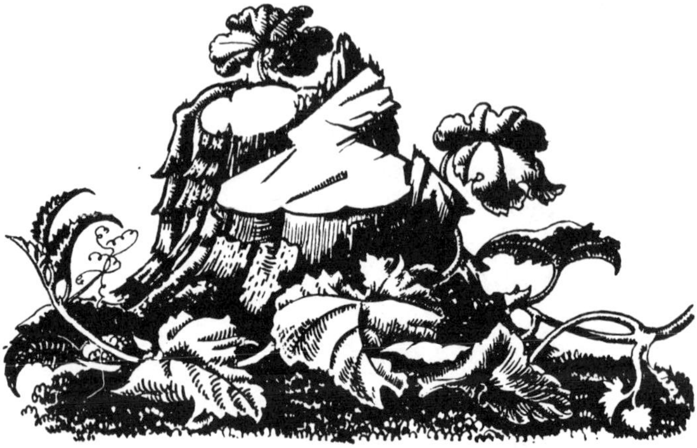

The Lord God Planted a Garden

Talking two rows at time, the midwives came to their meeting directly from the first Garden and Canning Fair at the Dunbar Colored School. They were full of talk about exhibits and prizes and they had to get some of the talk out of their systems before they could settle down to the business of learning how to operate an incubator for premature babies. The nurse had been too busy to go to the Fair, so they all wanted to tell her about it. For a few minutes everybody talked at once.

"I got the first prize for gourds," Aunt Jeanie announced before she was up the stairs. "The judges said they never saw such long, straight handles on dipper gourds nor such a heap of different kinds of other gourds. They all growed on my garden fence all around—"

Aunt Collie interrupted her to say, "My acorn squashes took a prize. They ain't bore none at all till just before the Fair they put out blooms and made these squashes that took the prize."

Then someone else broke in to tell how her tomatoes won a prize but her neighbor reminded her, "You got them out of Mis' Celia Foster's garden. I know for a fact you never raised nothing on your place 'sides cotton and a patch of sweet taters and a few rows of collards."

"I did too raise what I took to the garden show. I tended Mis' Celia's garden for her all summer. It was nearly 'bout same as mine."

Then to stop an argument the nurse asked who got the most prizes at the Fair. Everybody answered in the same breath, "Lou Della Foster—Lou Della Garland she is now—got the most prizes for garden stuff and for canned goods too."

"I knowed she was going to tote off prizes. I knowed it first time I looked over the fence at her garden this spring," Aunt Collie remembered. "There she was chopping away at the good straight rows of things, getting out every last little weed. Her little Nanette, three years old, was playing in the good clean garden dirt and wearing a leaf apron Lou Della made out of leaves from the chinaberry tree by the garden fence. The baby was standing up in a big cotton basket set in the shade. Now and again she took the baby out of the basket to rest it, and play with it and Nanette a little while. Her man's old uncle, Foolish John, was plowing their mule in the sweet tater patch."

"Us Foster colored folks always raised gardens—clear back to slavery times," Aunt Jeanie put in. "Old Colonel Foster learned us to do that, so we had plenty garden stuff long years before this war come on and the government started pushing people to make gardens. Colonel Foster said to my papa one day, 'Rome, you don't get no rest from your garden, do you? This damned climate keeps you gardening the whole year round.' Lou Della's got a green thumb like her great grandpa and a will to work like her great granny had—my papa and mama, you know," Aunt Jeanie said to the nurse.

"Lou Della is the youngest girl of Jeanie's nephew Jake," Aunt Collie added. "Jake is Mam Bob's boy, and Mam Bob is Jeanie's sister. With all their other children growed and married Jake and Rachel made over Lou Della a heap."

"In the family we always call her by her basket name, Ludy," Aunt Jeanie took up the story again. "It don't seem no time at all since the year before we got into this war, the year when Ludy and Hal picked cotton in the same cotton patches and done a lots of courting too. Hal's whole name is Hallelujah Garland. His mama named him right after she been to a camp meeting revival. But everybody calls him just plain Hal. Well, anyhow, Hal and Ludy sang and laughed and picked cotton with the rest of us and didn't care one bit if they got teased."

"I guess Hal helped Ludy to get her cotton sack full," the nurse said to Aunt Jeanie.

Aunt Jeanie just laughed, "I reckon not. Ludy could beat him; she was so quick. She could pick fifteen hundred pounds in a week without straining herself any bit—and sing and fun while she picked. White folks can't do that. Last year when the pickers were scarce the white folks's schools and business let out for them to pick cotton that never had in their lives done so. Mostly they tried hard but they got leaves and trash in the cotton they picked and never got much for theyselves but a misery in they back. One white lady said her back broke plumb in two and hung down behind and all day long she only picked thirty-five pounds. We ain't discriminating against white folks, but we don't want them in the same cotton field with us. Not because they're white but for a better reason. They spoil all the fun. Can't no white folks sing while they picking cotton. It's contrary to their nature.

"But to come back to Ludy and Hal. They'd pick cotton all day and then run and chase each other like they never done a lick of work—as we came home from the cotton patch. And they sang continuous and all the time.

"That was a good cotton year and folks had a little money to spend after they settled up their debts. Cotton market time folks start thinking, 'Who-all does I owe money to and who-all and how much is owing me?' You hear a heap of talk about foolish spending after cotton picking time, but mostly folks spends for things they has to have, or anyway for some things they wants mighty bad.

"Ludy got her some white slippers with part of her cotton picking money, though her mama tried to talk her out of it—being October like it was. But Ludy said she picked cotton special to buy them white slippers she wanted all her life—and a yellow dress. Mis' Celia let Ludy go to town with her and took her to the best store to buy her dress. If Ludy went by herself the clerks wouldn't show Ludy their best dresses in the store, for they didn't want their best trade to go to colored folks. But when Mis' Celia was along they were real polite about Ludy wanting a nice yellow dress that would fit good. Mis' Celia helped her pick out a little nothing of a green hat and a green pocketbook. And then she was all fixed up for Sunday, and a little money left to put in her green pocketbook.

"Hal had more money than Ludy, for he had a part interest in a bale of cotton he helped his daddy raise on their own ground. He bought himself a pearl gray felt hat and a pair of Sunday shoes. And then he spent himself big for a car—to finish up his courting in, he said. It was an old time car—what they called Molly T. It looked unstylish and made a lot of racket but it ran good. Hal come by Jake's on Saturday night to show Ludy the car and take her for a little ride. He said to be ready early to go to church the next day with him in his car.

"Same as always, church was along about two o'clock to give time for the women that cooked and served

Sunday dinner at white folks's houses. But Ludy was ready long ahead of the hour. Rachel, her mama, was ready too. It was big church meeting with a basket dinner. So Rachel packed her dinner in a washtub—all but her sugar pudding. Rachel didn't say nothing, but Ludy knowed her mama aimed to ride in the car with her and Hal. So when Hal drove up, she said she wasn't quite ready and would he take her mama on to church early. Her papa, Jake, would drive the mules to the wagon to take the washtub of dinner and for him and Rachel to ride back. Rachel is a big woman and she was tight squeezed into the back seat of that little car. Away she went, jouncing up and down with the sugar pudding on her lap. Ludy stood and watched them out of sight, not remembering it is bad luck to do that.

"When Hal got back to Ludy's house he put her in the front seat with him, and her looking as pretty as red shoes. They passed Jake on the road and waved to him. They got to church and rode some of their friends up and down in front of the church on the main crossroads. Then they went into the church service for a while to please their folks. They paid no mind to the preacher, though, but looked out the window at their car. Hal acted like he didn't hardly know whether to look at the car or a Ludy, they both looked so pretty to him.

"After the basket dinner they rode around some more. And then Hal stopped the car by the church and said, 'I got to see a man about six bits he owes me,' and he left Ludy sit in the car. The girls gathered round and asked a million questions. They said, 'Can you drive this car? I bet Hal won't let you.'

" 'Sure I can drive this car,' Ludy declared, though she never in her life tried to drive nothing more than Jake's old mules. 'How come he won't let me?' Ludy said to the girls gathered around. 'What makes you say that? To drive this car you just mash down on one thing and pull out another and twist the wheel around.'

"And to show how, Ludy suited the action to the words. Hal's little old Molly T took out across the cotton patch by the church, bumping over the cotton rows and making a track as crooked as a snake's trail in dog days. Folks lit out after the car, yelling at Ludy to stop. But she never knowed how to stop till the car got stuck in the wet sand on the bank of the river and stopped short to cough and shiver and then give up and set there sunk deep in the sand.

"They had to bring mules to pull the Molly T out and get it back to the church house. Then it wouldn't run by itself and the tires and wheels were all boogered up. Ludy sat in the car all that time to keep her white slippers clean. Jake and Rachel made her go home with them in the wagon, while Hal stayed with some men and boys by the church trying to fix his car.

"After they fixed on it till coming dark the car still wouldn't run, so they got in a crap game and Hal lost his car to another man. Then Hal got mixed up in a fight and got in jail and lay there overnight.

"Mr. Sterling Foster paid his fine and got Hal out of jail on Monday morning. He gave Hal a good going-over. 'Car gone. Cotton money wasted. Like as not, your girl done quit you.' Mr. Sterling said them things to Hal with all the details and particulars thrown in.

"Hal just said, 'It was a good car, Mr. Sterling, while it lasted. And I done resigned from gambling. And I hope Ludy ain't quit me.'

"His car *was* gone and his cotton money *was* wasted, but his girl hadn't quit him.

"Next Monday Hal and Ludy both came to see Mr. Sterling. Told him they got married Sunday while they both had good new clothes. They were looking for a place to live. Their mamas gave them some housekeeping things.

" 'Now we need a house and some ground to tend and somebody to furnish rations till next cotton picking time,' Hal explained to Mr. Sterling.

"He studied a while and then he had a proposition to make. 'Would you want to live in that little house down by Poison Lake that I built to stay in when I fish and hunt down there—only I never have time to fish nor hunt? It's a good little three room house with screens and a screened porch—and some of the heavy furniture like stoves and beds are there. I keep a big herd of cattle down there on that lowland pasture. If you will look after the cattle for me, you can live in the house free and I'll furnish rations for you. Then you can have clear whatever you can raise on the land you tend down there.'

"That sounded like a good bargain to Hal and Ludy and they took him up on it. They knowed old folks were afraid to stay down there since St. Paul got drowned in the lake, but they weren't afraid nowhere with each other.

"It was good rich land where they moved to—black swamp dirt. It was a lonesome land though. The trees grew tall and dark and the moss hung down from them long and gray. Owls sat on dead limbs and talked about dead things. But Hal and Ludy were as happy as song birds on a limb. They had a good house, and plenty rations and each other. They kept a team of Mr. Sterling's mules to haul feed and salt from town for the cattle. Every Saturday they had to make a trip to town to get feed for the cattle and their own rations. They stayed over Sunday with his folks or hers. And when folks asked them wasn't they afraid to go back to the lonesome swamps on Sunday night, they laughed and said they were so happy they broke the bad spell on Poison Lake and anybody could live there safe when they left.

"Soon there were brush heaps where Hal was cleaning the bushes away to make him some fields to plant. One Saturday after Christmas when folks started planting their early garden, Ludy started begging Mr. Sterling to furnish her some garden seeds. 'The Lord God planted a garden first thing when he set two young folks up to housekeeping on a rich piece of land. Garden of Eden he named it.' Mr. Sterling let her have five dollars to buy seeds with and I was in the store when she bought them—all kinds of vegetables and things.

"Then all summer long we heard tales about that

garden of hers when they came out from the swamps of a Saturday—the fine vegetables they had to eat and the things Ludy was canning up for wintertime. 'May have to dig a cellar or make a shed room or smokehouse to store things in we raised,' she said. 'Canned fruit and vegetables get in the way so bad in the house and I ain't started to can my tomatoes yet. Watermelons coming on and watermelon preserves to make—and goodness knows what all things.'

"Hal didn't brag none. He just said, when folks asked him, that he had a fine cotton crop and nice patches of corn and sweet taters. He left the garden talk to Ludy.

"Ludy was expecting a baby that summer and women folks warned her not to stand over the hot stove to can garden stuff. Some said no use for her to can anyhow. Stuff canned by a woman in her condition would spoil. Some said it wouldn't spoil only if she got too tired to can it good. Ludy said she knowed her canned goods won't spoil no matter what.

"When Hal came for me in late August to tend on Ludy when she birthed her baby, I thought to myself, 'Now I'll get to see that pretty garden and be the first to say how pretty it looks. Now I can count all that canned goods and tell my neighbors how many of all different kinds.'

"It was pitch black dark when we got there. They had a good little house with three rooms and Ludy had kept it nice. I didn't see no jars of canned goods on the shelves or under the beds. So I thinks, 'They got a cellar dug or a shed room built to keep it in.'

"After sunup, when the baby was birthed and dressed and Ludy had gone to sleep, I slipped out in the early morning for a breath of air and because I couldn't wait no longer to see that fine garden. I looked about and searched the place over. But the only sign of a garden I could find was one little squash vine growing around a stump—and it had come up volunteer without nobody planting it. I was so surprised that I felt like I turned a bird loose.

"All the two weeks I stayed there I never mentioned the garden and they never neither. I knowed how a woman do imagine things when she is expecting a baby—imagines things she don't feel like doing—imagines them till they come to be real in her mind.

"When folks asked me about Ludy's garden after I went home, I said, 'You have to see for yourself.' And the next year they did see. And it turned out fine as she told about it. Nobody but her and Hal and me ever knowed that first year's garden was one she conjured up in her mind but never planted into the ground.

"Even since that time, she's had the finest garden in the country. Last year just after cotton picking time Hal went to the war. She couldn't stay down there in the swamp by herself with a lap baby and a yard baby. They made good money down there raising cotton and garden stuff, and Ludy raised a cow from an orphan calf Mr. Sterling and Hal gave her.

"With the money her and Hal had saved they bought a mule and paid some on a house and some ground—near to other folks. Hal's old uncle, Foolish John, stays with Ludy and the babies and chops the wood and tends the cow and plows the mule. Ludy gets army allotment from the government and pays on their property. She keeps her and the babies and Foolish John with rations and clothes, but she don't waste none of her government money. And she keeps her house clean and raises a fine garden.

"Mr. Sterling was a judge at the Fair today and so he saw all the colored folks' fine garden stuff and canned rations. And he said, 'Looks like you folks fixed up good for winter rations.' Then he saw all them things of Ludy's with prize ribbons and he said to her, 'Looks like the Lord God planted a garden on your place, Lou Della. You couldn't win all these prizes by yourself. You had a fine garden, though, ever since you been married, ain't you?'

"Ludy just said, 'Yes, sir, Mr. Sterling,' to him; but she turned around and winked at me and I knowed her and me together was remembering that lone little squash vine growing around a stump."

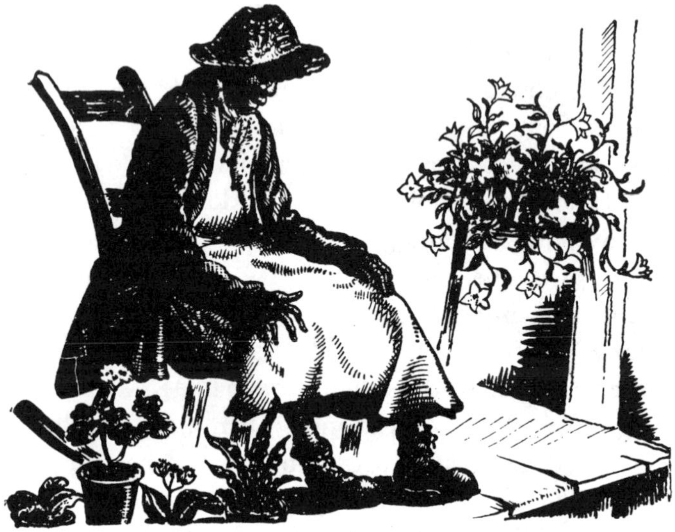

The Pink of the Evening

"YOU looking for Aunt Dilly?" one of her neighbors asked as I walked through the colored section of a little county seat town in South Georgia. "Yes'm, I reckon she's home or maybe across the street where the folks are waiting for a funeral. You be surprised how young Aunt Dilly's getting. Calls herself working out, her going on eighty-eight years old."

Sure enough, Aunt Dilly was at home, sitting on her front porch in the sunshine of a February afternoon. But, as she said, she was "as good as across the street," for she was quite occupied with watching the crowd gather for the funeral. And until the funeral crowd moved on to the church, her talk was concerned with the people arriving across the street. "Look at that purple suit now. Like as not she gets war allotment money and puts it all on her back. Can you see the hearse coming to bring him for the funeral? Heathen way to do, sending a person off to the undertakers to get fixed for the funeral and nobody sitting up with his corpse at night. There goes his white folks to pay their respects with some flowers. Their folks as good as raised him. Yes'm, he was older than me. Past ninety and used to brag how he would live to be a hundred. But the Lord didn't let him. It don't pay to brag in the face of the Almighty how long you aim to live. I gave all my flowers in bloom to dress the church for the funeral—all but my camellias. I kept them on the bushes for me and my friends to look at."

Finally the funeral moved on to the church and Aunt Dilly was ready to talk about herself. She had invited me to come because she said the Lord had viewed her to tell me about her life. She talked all that afternoon and three days thereafter. To make this chapter it has been a matter of picking and choosing from the revelations of those three and a half days of conversation.

Aunt Dilly began with genealogy as autobiographers so often do. "On my mother's side we can trace back to my great great granny. On my father's side just back to him. You know in slavery times the mother's side of a colored child's family was the side that was sure and certain—just in the nature of things. My mama's folks had been with the same family since great granny's day. They lived on a plantation seven miles outside this town. My father came from Roanoke, Virginia, where our master went and bought him and some more slaves and brought back home with him. His name was Charlie and after the war when colored people had to have two names he took the last name of the folks that owned him, for that name would give him better connections.

"My mama had three children before he lived with her and then she had ten with him—thirteen in all. Her two oldest children got sold away from her and she never heard tell of them no more. All her life long her heart grieved to hear even as little as was they dead or alive—but never a word. She said over and over from her heart that was the worst thing to a woman about slavery, to be haunted with fear that your children would be sold away and separated from you forever more. And she had that fear multiplied thirteen times over in her soul, for she never had a child born free. Though she longed to know how it would feel to birth a child in freedom.

"Some years before the war in the time of emancipation, some years before freedom, folks came through the country in secret, stirring up the colored people to run away to freedom in the North country. And my daddy wanted to run away in the night and make ourselves free. But Mama said, 'How far you think I get with all this pack of children? We get caught before we get started good. Anyhow, I don't know how I'd feed my children up in the North country where I ain't got us no white connections.'

"Then one dark night my daddy just took his foot in his hand and ran off and left Mama and her children behind. They got along about as well without him, I reckon, but Mama was lonesome. She wouldn't have no other man in her cabin. After about a year my daddy slipped back. He was that fond of Mama, and he got wore out with hiding and not knowing which way to turn. He hid around for a long time and stayed with Mama all he could without getting caught. Mama did fine laundry for the ladies at the plantation house. And one day they noticed her shape and said to her, 'I'm glad you forgot that runaway Charlie and took you another man.'

"And Mama said, 'This ain't no other man's child but Charlie's.' So they found him. And that child was me.

"I don't remember the war much except all the people being hungry and scared such a long time. This ground wasn't fought over, though the fighting got close to here.

"After the war and freedom a lots of people, white and colored—mostly colored, for they always been more than half the people in this county—moved off to other places to make a new start. The white folks had lost what they had and the colored folks had got their freedom. During and after all the wars in my time there's been a great moving out from this county to other places where people thought they could better theyselves. After the emancipation war the colored people here had the fever to go to Oklahoma, and great swarms of them went there, though some drifted back.

"My daddy was all in a swivet to go, but Mama said, No, she couldn't go. She lived through the war with her family of children safe and alive and now she wouldn't take them to Oklahoma to get killed with the Indians. That made him mad and he went off and lay about town for a week drinking mean whisky. Then he came back to help Mama raise the children. Some years later he went off and died way down in Mississippi. Mama said he wouldn't rest comfortable in heaven 'less he could travel to its four corners now and again.

"I took a husband when I was fourteen years old, and I had thirteen children too, like Mama. And they all lived to be grown. I got only four living now, a girl living here in this town and a boy out in the county. Then I got a girl in Jersey City and a boy in a big city close to her—that's my youngest boy, going on fifty-seven years old. One of my boys died in the last war before this one with foreign countries. In the time of that war and right after it was when business was good and jobs a-plenty up North and all my children but the two that still lives here went up North to work and lived there ever since. Not all in the same cities, though. Most of them died up there. It's an unhealthy climate to change to from here and from outdoors work here to inside jobs mostly—and in winter the air is pure ice and lungs trained to breathe down here just clog up and break down with breathing in ice all winter long —and I mean *long*. The young generation raised there gets used to it I reckon, for my grandchildren and great grands don't die off with t.b. and pneumonia and other lung diseases like my children did.

"I went up there to visit once but I didn't like it. I loved to see my children but they didn't live as good as I thought they would with cash wages through the year. They lived in houses with other people, apartments they call them, crowded up in ugly parts of town. No porches to sit on, no room to plant things, and factory dirt all over things. But they do make good wages and they got some privileges, like voting in elections and such things.

"They wouldn't let me work. Just wanted me to sit there till they got home from work. Nobody for me to visit with but them. They wouldn't let me go nowhere by myself for fear I'd get lost in the city. The things to eat were different and not to my taste. They wanted me to sell my place down here and stay with them. They said they'd even get me fixed up to vote. Now I'm proud to see my own children and grandbabies vote, but I'm too old to take politics on my shoulders in a strange part of the country. Down here where I know all the people I'd love to vote once in a while for a good man I like. But voting away from home would be doing things with my eyes shut.

"And my church is down here where I taught Sunday School for forty-nine years. When I was school age the colored people here had two months' school in a year.

Now the colored high school in this town has nine months in a year. But I learned to read right good, though I don't write much but my sign name. Mostly I read my church papers and Sunday School books. My grandchildren send me colored people's newspapers but mostly I give them away to young folks to read. Mostly they're meant for them that are striving upward to more rights and things. And me, I'm too old and lived too long to strive upward to anything but heaven. So I read my church reading that heads me in that direction.

"And so I came back home from my visit before Christmas. I like to be where my friends are. My children and grandchildren follow their own minds and have their friends. And they ain't same as mine. And I wanted to start my year's work between the Christmases —old and new Christmas—for luck in the year's undertakings.

"And some folks down here were depending on me, for I was then a granny-midwife. The Lord laid that burden on my shoulders when I was forty years old and I toted the burden faithful till He viewed me to lay it down when I was going on eighty. The nurses said I needed a rest and so I asked the Lord to show me what to do. And he viewed me to give up my license and my bag of midwife things and step down off the Board. So the nurses and the midwife club had a ceremony for me and gave me my purple and gold badge with the seal of Georgia and Retired Midwife on it in gold and my name on the pin that fastens it to my clothes. No, they didn't give it to me, either. They said I earned it. And when I wear it I leave my coat open.

"My grandmother was a midwife but not my mama. I learned from doctors and from going with older midwives before I started on my own. There weren't no licenses then, nor no blood tests to see if people's blood was moral, nor no birth certificates. No connection of the midwife and her business with the Law and the government. A lots of the grannies had a dread of the new way with Law wound up in it but it turned out good.

"The birth records are one good thing. It don't leave everything hung on our memory. It's there on the Law books who was born and when and to what people for parents.

"Now that I don't practice no more some women that I tended other times wants me to come and just be there to make them feel good. One woman that I caught nine good healthy babies for wanted me to come and just lay my hands on her with the last one coming. It made her feel better, she said, if I touched her. I never caught but one white baby in all the years. And I wasn't proud of that, for the mother had a mighty bad name, but somebody had to go to the poor woman. And the Lord frowns on folks that scorn human misery.

"Now I got a little pension for old age and I got my house we bought forty-five years ago—a pretty good house yet. I rent a room to a school teacher, and another to an old man with no home, and I cook for a boy that tends my flowers and garden. I work out a little, staying with children of nights till their parents come home. I got my insurance to put me away nice when I die—whenever that may be. But I ain't in no hurry to go. Heaven's my home but I ain't homesick yet. I like to have some time to sit on my own front porch and enjoy the pink of the evening with my friends passing by, and my flowers about me, and the burdens of years behind me.

"When I sit here remembering the years behind me, one of the prettiest times to recollect is my wedding. You know in slavery times colored people didn't marry with courthouse papers and all that. When me and my husband took each other to live with, the times weren't many years past the ways of slavery times. We lived faithful and decent together and papers to say we belonged married to each other were a thing we never bothered with. Then when some of our children were grown and others little yet, the oldest girls wanted us to be married proper with papers that came from the Law. Their daddy was a hard person to talk into it, for he saw no reason in what the girls wanted us to do. But I know how young folks want things about their parents so they can be proud and not behind the times. So I begged their daddy into getting the license for us. Maybe it seemed funny to some—but to me it was the prettiest time of my life. I was just a little past thirty and young in my heart for nice occasions. My white family gave me the new white dress and meeting drops in a pretty glass bottle and washtubs of roses off their fences full of climbing roses. And all my friends were nice to me and made everything pretty for the occasion. My mama said a bride not a virgin should wear some purple on her wedding day. So I had a wide purple sash on my white dress. Any woman, whatever color she is, belongs to have a pretty wedding no matter if it comes soon or late.

"The other time I get most pleasure to remember is when I went to the circus and saw all the strange sights and animals that were named as going in the ark in old Noah's day. It was when I was ten years old the circus came to this town the first time. Weeks on end people talked about it. When the day came my daddy slipped off to town with the youngest in our family to the circus. I was drove off to school where it was a misery to go with a circus in town. It was more misery than I could bear and so I ran away from school and walked the seven miles to town and found the circus. I didn't know it cost money to get in and I broke down completely when they wouldn't let me in without money. Then a kind person—to this day I don't know if it was man or woman—took me in to see the wonders of the circus. Never could I find words to tell about it. Even today after all these years when I aim to tell you all about it, the wonder of it rises up in me and stops the words from coming. And so I just sit here on the porch in the pink of the evening and remember."

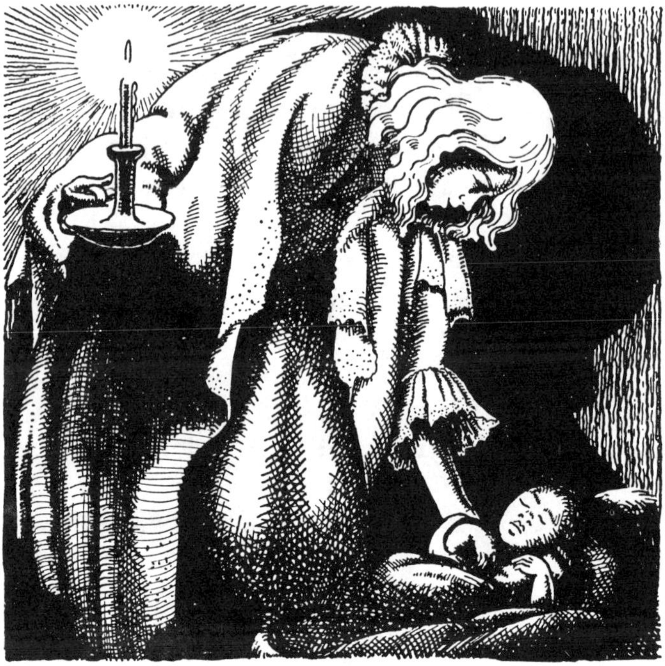

I Learned Some Latin

"SPEAKING of learning things," said Aunt Dilly as we sat on her porch watching the children going home from school, "speaking of learning things, old as I am, I learned some Latin a few years back. I learned it thoroughly good, too, and I can still say it. I needed to know some Latin, and seeing as how I had learned a lots of things from the nurses, I just asked the health nurse if she could learn me a few words.

" 'Whatever do you want to know Latin for, Aunt Dilly?' she asked me. She was going home from her work and had come by my house for some camellias I had promised her. So she sat down on my porch while I told her for what purpose I needed to know Latin.

" 'It's to lay a ghost,' I told her.

"And she said, 'Well, I've done a lot of things in my day but I never helped lay a ghost. Go ahead and tell me about it. I think I could teach you some Latin words if that's all it takes to get rid of this ghost, but I'd like to hear about it first.'

" 'Well,' I said, 'somebody told me that they read in a book or heard somehow about saying Latin to a ghost. That sounds proper for this ghost I'm talking to you about, for it is an educated ghost.

"Do you remember that old house with the wide lawn and big trees and the old flower garden gone wild out on the Pike? That's the place where this ghost lived. It's Mis' Rose's ghost. Her name was Madonna Rose but we always called her Mis' Rose. The house used to be her home, though she's been dead some twenty years. Her family were my family's white folks, so I know all about her.

"When she was young she married her lover when he was on his deathbed. He begged her to bear his name through life, so she put on all her wedding finery and married him while he lay there sick. Then she put back on her everyday clothes and nursed him till he died three days after the wedding. She put on deep black mourning and stayed close at home for two whole years. Then she took off all her mourning, all but a mourning ring she wore above her wedding ring and a cameo pin of her lover's likeness set in black enamel with little pearls circled around. Them two mourning jewels she wore to the day of her death—even wore them when she was asleep. She pinned the cameo on her nightdress every night and never took off the rings except to bathe herself.

"After she laid aside her mourning, she went to the city and bought three trunks full of new clothes and went to teach in a stylish school for young ladies. She didn't have to do that for the pay, because her family were people of means and she inherited her husband's money and property. She said she just wanted to be useful in life.

"She had a fine education with all the extra things it was stylish for young ladies to be educated in, like music and foreign tongues and fine needlework and painting on china. She was dainty and sweet and so pretty the men just swarmed around her any time she came out in society. My mama and me talked about it and we thought it was a sad waste to shut herself up in that school and stay a widow when she loved children and had such a fine sense of home. Mama said Mis' Rose, for all her being dainty and refined, could have a dozen children and never mind a bit nor lose her good looks neither. Sometimes I wish Mama had spoke her mind to Mis' Rose and tried to keep her from being so faithful to a dead man and toting his name through life.

"For years Mis' Rose stayed at the young ladies' school. Then a few years before she was fifty she came back here and made her house and garden and a place to call home. Hers wasn't the biggest nor the finest place around here, but it was the prettiest and the homiest. It was pure magic how that lone woman could give a house such a home feeling about itself. Colored folks loved to work there—mostly my people. My mama and me did her fine laundry; my husband kept the grounds as long as she lived. Me and my girls have worked there, and through the years her cook was always from my kin people. She had a nice care for home living and wanted things done right, but she wasn't never cranky. I remember how she used to count the silver late at night when she was dressed for bed with a dressing gown over her nightdress, and then go all over the house with a candle in her hand to see if things were in proper order.

"Always she had some niece or nephew in the house and in summer the house was full of children and young people. She was a power for good in the neighborhood with building up schools and other common good. Mostly other people got the credit, because she didn't want to be made public. She helped me a lots with clothes and things for babies of women I tended as granny-midwife. Fine dainty baby clothes that she sewed herself and nice food and things for the mother. She used to give me such things for them that needed.

"Her own clothes were the prettiest I ever saw. After the corsets and formal attire in that school where she had lived for years, she wore loose robes a lot in the privacy of her own house. Morning wrappers of blue silk mull, or white challis with pink rosebuds, or white India linen with lace and ribbons, or pale yellow lawn with hamburg embroidery. Mama and me loved to wash and iron them. Later in the day or at night—any time after morning when she wasn't dressed formal—she wore rich dressing gowns over her petticoats or her nightdress. Rich green brocade, bronze satin, rose color watered silk, white taffeta with violets. In such flowing rich robes she was the most beautiful—enough to tempt a man out of his senses, only no man ever saw her dressed like that. Her petticoats and underdrawers were all fine with lace and embroidery. Mama used to say, 'Ain't it a shame nobody ever sees these lacy underthings but her washerwoman and her maid?' When clothes got plain and skimpy, Mis' Rose kept right on wearing what suited her style, though folks called her old-fashion.

"When she was close to eighty, she died. They buried her by her young husband, and put her name on his sad rock. For some years she rested quiet in her grave. Then her spirit began to walk the earth as a troubled spirit will.

"She had willed her house and other property to twenty nieces and nephews. To be sure, they divided up the money and spent it in whatever direction they pleased. But when it came to the house the division was a hard matter. Some wanted the house for themselves, some wanted the money out of it. Some wanted one thing, some another. Not all of them would ever agree to sell out to any one of them that wanted the house. They couldn't make up their minds to sell it outside the family. They took the furnishings and divided and quarreled over them. But after some twenty years them nieces and nephews and their heirs still owned the house together.

"For a long time it stood empty. Then they started to rent it out. And you know how a house goes to neglect in them circumstances. Mama used to say Mis' Rose ought to come back and haunt people if they didn't take nice care of her place after she was gone. Well, about ten years ago people started seeing Mis' Rose at night, going about the house with her candle and wearing her rich, pretty dressing gowns the way she had done in life. It was just women that saw her, for Mis' Rose's ghost in a dressing gown would never show itself to a man. The colored people that knew her so good in life saw her first. Of course she never bothered nobody, but it made some people uneasy to live there.

"I used to see her myself when I went there, mostly when folks in the house had a new baby. No, I never was scared of Mis' Rose's ghost. I said to myself, 'Her poor spirit is troubled over the way her earthly home is going to ruin and she comes here at night to look through the house the way she did in life.' It bothered me for her sweet soul not to have its proper rest. So I thought of ways to lay her ghost and keep her spirit in untroubled rest. That was when I asked the nurse to help me learn some Latin.

"And she said, 'Well, I studied Latin in school but I remember better some of the Latin poetry my father used to say to us. He was a doctor and he liked a Latin verse that was a joke about a man that felt a little bit bad and called a doctor that gave him chills and fever and made him bad sick.' So she learned me to say in Latin:

> Languebam sed tu comitatus protinus ad me
> Venisti centum, Symmache, discipulis;
> Centum me tetigere manus aquilone gelatae;
> Non habui febrem Symmache, nunc habeo.

"Right soon after I learned that Latin there was a new baby at Mis' Rose's house. And there in the middle of the night with everybody asleep but me, for the baby had come and the mother dozed off, there came Mis' Rose with her candle and stood over the new baby. It was a summer night and she had on her cool white taffeta dressing gown with the purple violets sprinkled thick over it. But she looked young again—not old like when she died. I got up my nerve and said the Latin verse to her with my eyes shut, thinking when I opened them her spirit would be gone to eternal rest never more to walk the earth. But when I looked again there she was plain as life standing by me. And it was just like speaking to her in life.

" 'Don't be troubled over no house,' I said to her. 'Earthly houses don't make no difference to you no more. Leave this old house go and take your long rest in heavenly mansions.'

"Then she told me what brought her spirit back to her home on earth. 'I don't have a care for the house,' she told me. 'It's the babies in the house that carry me back here to watch in the night. All my life long I was starved for little babies of my own in my own house. So now I watch over other people's babies in my house. That's all I can do, for I've lived my life already and can't make it different now.'

"Then I said to Mis' Rose, 'But this is a little colored baby you're watching over now.'

" 'Color don't have any connection with people up where I come from tonight,' she said to me. And I got to thinking how heaven wouldn't have no color line. When I came back out of my deep thoughts, Mis' Rose was gone. She was seen again after that from time to time. Sometimes she talked to me, sometimes not. I never tried no more to drive her away with Latin. With thirteen babies of my own in my lifetime I couldn't have the heart to deny the spirit of a woman that hungered for babies all her life and even after her life was done.

"Then one stormy dark night Mis' Rose was seen in her house for the last time. Early in the night she went from room to room with her candle. Late in the night the house burned down. Some said it was struck by lightning and caught on fire. Some said the fire caught from Mis' Rose's candle. Nobody could ever remember carrying the two babies out of the burning house, but there they were safe and sound wrapped warm in their blankets and lying by the garden gate. It was lucky for them that Mis' Rose chose to come that night. No doubt but she laid them there safe and then went back to her eternal rest for evermore."

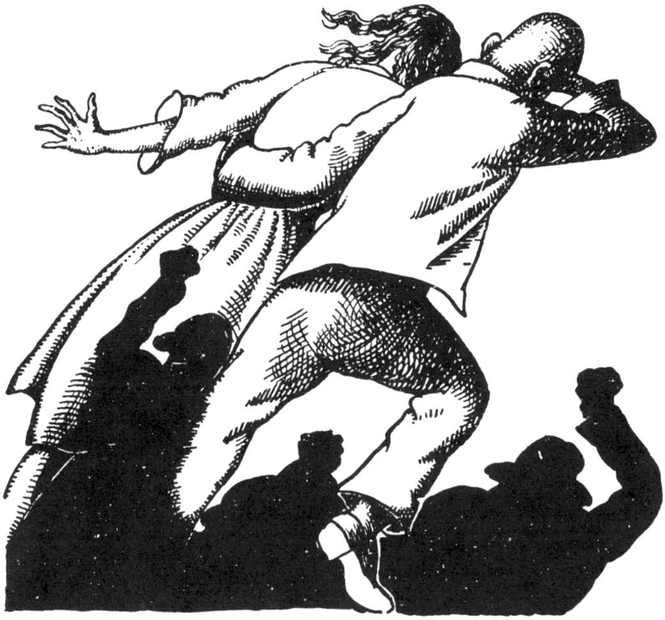

Gift Child

THIS story does not come from the sociable talk of midwives meeting together. It comes from intimate conversation of two friends of different races. It is told here because Mam Bob wants one of her stories written, and this is what she chooses to tell and the way she chooses to tell it:

"It is an old story—as old as sorrow—but it is new again when it happens to one of your own. This happened to our gift child that came to us because my sister was a granny-midwife. We gave our gift child the basket name of Pet, for that is what she was to all us folks in the family. And that is what we always called her.

"We knew all about Pet's folks that she came from to us, because our great-aunty helped birth her grandmother, our aunty her mother, and my sister Jeanie tended Pet's mother when she birthed her. Pat's grandmother on her mother's side was a free issue Negro—the word for a person with a white mother and colored man for a father. To people's minds that is a lots worse than a colored mother and a white father. No, I can't tell you why it is. Jesus knows I don't know. But that is the way people think about it.

"When her baby was still young, folks in the neighborhood ran the white mother and her baby's father out of the county. We heard afterwards that they went down on the coast and caught the yellow fever and died together. They wanted to take the baby with them but the crowd that chased them out of the county—white and colored folks too in the crowd—wouldn't let them take the baby.

"They weren't mean people. The worst thing against them was this free issue child. The man's old granny raised the baby. Lots of folks scorned her on account of her mother. But she grew to be a nice woman and married a good mulatto man. Then she died when her baby was little and that was Pet's mother. She married a light-skinned man too, and Pet was for the world like a white child without a taint of color that showed in any way at all. Her daddy swore at first that he believed she was a white man's child, but the mother said she wasn't, and that was the truth. Sister Jeanie and me knew her well, and she didn't have no white man's child. We been going in and out of the back doors of people's houses all our lives and sometimes the back doors of people's minds too. And we can sort out the liars and the hypocrites, and to our best knowledge Pet's mother told the truth. All the white blood in her and her man got together and made a white child, and that's all there was to it.

"The mother died in a few months with some kind of fever and the father got killed with a train. There wasn't any close kin to take the baby to raise. Jeanie brought it to my house till we could find some place to make it a home. In a few days we loved it so good we couldn't bear to part from it, so we kept it for our gift child. My husband had a soft heart for orphan children, for he was a gift child himself, when his mother just slipped off and left him . . . but that story I'll tell you another time. This is Pet's story I'm telling now.

"We loved that baby so much we got plumb foolish about it. My youngest was fourteen, and it was a good feeling for all of us to have a little baby in the family again. Hannah was sixteen and she waited on the baby like a little mother. It was her that named it Anginora. When she went off to school the next year, she couldn't hardly bear to part from the baby.

"Mis' Celia, the white lady I cooked for—and my

mother and her mother before us cooked for different generations of the same family—she gave us things for the baby, a little bed and other things her children now grown and gone had used. And for a matter of a few years we were happy and untroubled about our gift child. Then the year before she started to school a thing happened that changed the feeling of things for all of us, but worst of all for Pet.

"Now and again I went to town on Saturdays with Mis' Celia and took Pet with me. That time we were waiting for her husband to come to start back home—her on the front seat, me and Pet on the back. Then one of her friends came along with a stranger and introduced him to Mis' Celia. He talked a while and when he turned to leave he said to Mis' Celia, 'You got a mighty pretty little girl sitting back there so quiet with her nurse.'

"Mis' Celia just said, 'Pet *is* a pretty child.'

"After the stranger was gone Mis' Celia's friend turned on her and stormed at her, 'Celia Foster, are you crazy! Letting anybody think that Negro child is yours! I'm ashamed and humiliated. Why didn't you tell him it was a Negro?' Then she got so mad her words ran together.

"Mis' Celia just said, 'I didn't want to hurt the child's feelings nor Mam Bob's.'

" 'A Negro's feelings!' her friend fairly screamed. 'I give up!' and she flounced away.

"Right soon we started back home. All the way there slow tears slid down on Mis' Celia's dress. And little Pet huddled to me like a scared creature hiding from harm. We never talked about it, but after that me and Pet never rode with Mis' Celia to town any more. She asked us many a time. But I couldn't be the cause of humbling a person before her friends after she humbled herself to save my child's feelings.

"After that it was never the same again with Pet. That was when she found out that she was a white child that had to be black. It was like somebody had hung a sign on her that said COLORED, stooping her heart to shame. Then my husband and me came to feel and know what a heavy duty we laid on our own shoulders to try to raise a white child to be black. My husband was an educated man and a good father to his own children, but this was beyond his wisdom. Myself, I had raised my own five children and helped our white folks some ways to raise theirs. But I raised my black children to be black and the white children to be white. That was the pattern to follow. But the knowledge of color didn't come so soon nor so ugly to my own children as to Pet. My own children so far as I know had no taint of white blood in them. We are colored people but we are proud colored people. We always had a good name and been respected for what we are by white folks and colored folks. We never suffered the miseries of some colored folks. We lived good with plenty to eat and had our own place to live, though we have worked for the same white folks on the plantation for generations back on my side. We sent our children off to school to be educated and to further their ambition.

So we could raise another child reasonable well so far as *things* went. But we didn't know how to ring the bells of freedom for a white child whose spirit was in bondage to the colored blood folks knew she had in her.

"She was a good child and so pretty it made your eyes hurt. And smart too. At school she learned to read a book and to back a letter sooner than any of our own children had. But she was a sad little thing. She loved us but she was not among us. She was all alone by herself in that wide place that lays between white and colored.

"About that time our youngest daughter died and we took her little boy Sterling to raise. This little black baby made a bright pattern of laughter among us but our little white child and her quiet sad ways were like the Songs of Sorrow.

"For a long time my husband and me could not name the thing nor talk about it. But there came a day when we said to each other that we would see if any way could be managed for her to be raised a white child from then on. We talked it out with ourselves and then we talked with Mis' Celia and Mr. Sterling. They helped us at times with our own children. But they said they didn't know any way at all to manage what we talked about, least ways where folks knew Pet had colored blood.

"That gave us a thought that maybe an orphan's home up North would take her for a white child. Two of our married daughters lived in two different big cities in the North. So my husband and Hannah took

Pet to visit one of our daughters. And then they went to an orphan's home with Pet to see if they would take and raise her for a white child. But they said no, they wouldn't fool people about her color. They talked reasonable and kind, but they said the rules were against it and people's minds and feelings were against it.

"So they brought Pet back home with them. She changed her name from Anginora because she said that sounded too much like a Negro name. She hid from people in mixed crowds so they wouldn't think she was white and then make a big to-do when they found out their mistake. Going to church or to town, as we rode along sitting in our chairs in the wagon, she held the parasol close to her body to cover her up when people passed by. It was like being colored put all joy beyond her reach on earth. And being white, she couldn't bend her spirit to white people. And it stabbed our love for her to our hearts.

"Then we sent her to live with my daughter—the one without children—where she could go to school with white children. It was our smothered hope that she could grow happy there. For a time she was happy, and then it all broke up around her. We didn't know, but she had let on she was a white child and nobody knew better till what they call a visiting teacher came to my daughter's house and found out the family was colored. And she went back and told it around. Pet might of got along all right there if she had been her true self. But the teachers and the children didn't like her for fooling them, and in the shame of it Pet couldn't get up spirit to go back there no more.

"We brought her back home and she went to school here till she was nearly about fourteen. We'll just pass over what happened in them years. And then we sent her to the other daughter's up North to go to high school with mixed children. My husband had died in that time and it lay on my shoulders to guide her. Before she went away I talked to her as a woman among women and told her she couldn't pass for a white person till she was old enough and knowledgeable enough to get along by herself without us forever. Till then she needed to stay with us and get educated and learn the ways of white folks every chance she had so she wouldn't give herself away when she left us. We didn't say the words 'cross the color line' but she knew and I knew that was a compelling thing in her heart and mind. When she came home of summers I kept her with me when I was at Mis' Celia's house and she worked with me and watched how things were fixed and how things were done nice in a white lady's home. Then after high school, she worked in my daughter's city and went to school of nights to learn more while she got older and more knowledgeable to take care of herself.

"Then came the time—when nor where nor how ain't mine to tell nor yours to know. But there came the time when in a far away city she found her place among her own people, and we never could any more lay the least claim to her. She had to lose herself to us in our family and to us in our race. For the sweet privilege of being a white woman she had to be alone in her knowledge of herself. And she had to be alone in her fears that some day in her life's span that somebody would find out she had a taint of color in her blood and tear her world apart. It is a hard thing for a woman's mind and spirit to be all times afraid and all times alone in fear—fear of her own color, fear her children will show color, fear unnamed for what it is —and nobody on the earth she so much as dare tell her fears to. That is a high price for any woman to pay for the sweet privilege of being white. And the burden of it makes black patterns of pain for her on my heart and mind. But I take a little comfort sometimes in knowing that the color she fears in herself will help her to bear it through life. For her colored blood can give her the deep patience to endure of colored people—a patience as old and as deep as our sorrow."

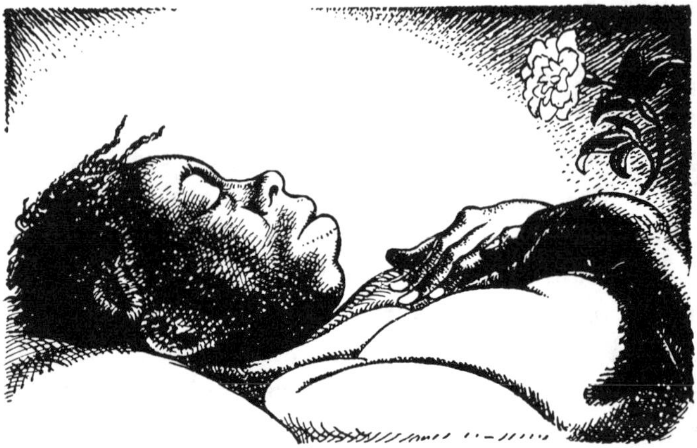

After a Little Rest

"'AFTER a little rest,' that's what she said. 'After a little rest, I'll come right back here to take hold and help out with sick folks and babies.' Aunt Charity was talking about Aunt Jeanie, who had been her dearest friend for years and on whom she depended for help and strength in many things, but especially in her work as a granny-midwife.

"I had been to Aunt Jeanie's for a visit that day," Aunt Charity went on as she settled down to her story. "And I had come out on the front porch to sit and wait for Jake to pass by in his wagon and carry me home on his way past my house. Aunt Jeanie was doing the last minute little things a woman person always does when she is leaving home for a visit off some place.

"Her niece, Hannah—Mam Bob's daughter, you know—had come over to hear Aunt Jeanie's instructions about how to take care of her live property around the place. There was the pig in the pen back of the garden, the guinea fowls, the biddies and the old frizzle-legged hen that was wanting to set, and the gray cat with kittens in the woodshed. Hannah didn't need all them instructions, for she had waited on Aunt Jeanie's property for years when Aunt Jeanie was grannying or when she was staying with folks to nurse their babies. But Hannah loved her auntie and loved to hear how thoughted she was for things that belonged to her.

"I could hear them talking in back of the house. And then they came around to the front porch for Hannah to look at the potted plants and get instructions about them.

" 'Now when that white geranium blooms out good,' Aunt Jeanie told her, 'I'd love for you to take it over to my old white friend, Grandma Ellis. She does love white flowers so, and her kin people are right neglectful about bringing her pretties. Seems like folks get neglectful about things that lift a sick body's spirits when the sickness goes along for years. And when the lavender blooms out just right, I'd love for you to dry some for me to put with my Sunday things to scent them up good.'

" 'And what about your gourds, Aunt Jeanie?' Hannah asked, noticing the fine gourds hanging on the gourd vines that climbed over and around the garden fence.

" 'Well,' said Aunt Jeanie, 'if I don't get back home before the Garden and Canning Fair, put them in with my name on them. I'd dearly love to take a prize this year like last for my gourds.'

"Hannah went around the house to gather the eggs and then go home so she could cook supper for the folks she worked for—where women in her family had cooked for generations. Aunt Jeanie brought in her chamber pot from the back yard picket fence where she hung it upside down to sun every morning after she had scalded it out with boiling hot water. Then she went in the house and busied about, putting the last little things in her suit satchel. I moved over close to the front door so I could still watch for Jake and see and talk with her too.

"She tried on her hats a lots of times in front of the looking glass, making up her mind which one to wear on her trip. Her mind settled on the little purple hat with a feather and she fastened it on with a hatpin. Then she put the rest of the hats in a hatbox to carry along. Not that she needed all them hats special, but she had always thought it was a mark of a lady to travel with a hatbox full of extra hats for different occasions. The white friend that she was going home with for a visit gave her the hatbox all new and Aunt Jeanie managed for the hats. The white lady said she loved to think about Aunt Jeanie feeling like a lady with a hatbox full of different hats to choose from.

"With her hat on, Aunt Jeanie thought about her cape jasmine bush and went out to pick the flowers of its late August blooming. She loved that flower bush, though cape jasmines are common as dirt, growing every place—in the gardens at the plantations, in the yards of Negro cabins, in the graveyards, and strayed along the roadsides where old houses had burned down. But no matter how plenty and common they were, Aunt Jeanie treasured them up. This time she picked every flower and every bud that showed a little streak of white. She packed them away with wet cotton in the box her new shoes came in and covered them over with silk paper and tied it all up with string to carry with her on her trip north, way into the upper part of Georgia where maybe the cape jasmines didn't bloom late into the summer and fall.

"Then her white friend that she aimed to visit with came by with Mr. Sterling to take them to catch a bus. And they said they would wait a little for Jake to come, because Mr. Sterling wanted to see him anyhow.

"That was when I told Aunt Jeanie I shore would miss her and I hoped she would get back home before Ludy's third baby came, because Ludy hadn't been so well as common and Aunt Jeanie had waited on her other times and knew the ways of her birthing. This time Ludy had spoke for me to wait on her because Aunt Jeanie had stepped down off the Board and didn't catch babies no more. But she would go in a case of need and stay close by and lend her strength of heart and mind to the granny-midwife and the mother birthing the baby. And, old as she was, she still went to help with sick folks around the neighborhood, whatever the nature of their misery and complaint. That was the reason why I said what I did.

"And Aunt Jeanie said, 'After a little rest' and told me how she was going home with her friend to rest a little while. It wasn't uncommon for Aunt Jeanie to visit her white folks. In a lots of the white folks' homes where folks knew her for her care of sick people and babies, she was welcome to visit even when they never had no sick people and didn't need no granny for a birthing.

"But her white friend laughed when Aunt Jeanie said, 'Rest awhile.' She said Aunt Jeanie got busy looking after her the minute they got to her house. 'I verily believe,' she declared, 'that Aunt Jeanie conjured me into having malaria last spring just because she loves to wait on sick people.'

" 'You hush your mouth, honey,' Aunt Jeanie said. 'You know you got that malaria fever prowling about the Georgia sea islands. And I ain't no conjure woman. And my folks here, black and white too, knows I rest up when I go to your house and they want me to go, they do.'

"Then Jake came along. And he put Aunt Jeanie's suit satchel and her hatbox in Mr. Sterling's car and we all left Aunt Jeanie's house, going different directions.

"When Aunt Jeanie and her friend got on the bus—so folks has told me—the bus driver was kind and let the colored people get on first and fill up their share of seats in the back of the bus, so they wouldn't have to scrouge past everybody the way they have to if they get on the bus last. A colored preacher moved over to let Aunt Jeanie sit next to the window so she could talk to her town friends outside till the bus started. It was a Wednesday and they were talking about going to prayer meeting that night.

" 'We wish you could go to prayer meeting with us,' they said to Aunt Jeanie. 'It would do your old heart good.'

" 'That it would, I know,' Aunt Jeanie agreed with them. 'But I never have been to prayer meetings much in my lifetime. If I went to the prayer meeting place, seemed like I always got called out—before the meeting got started most times. Somebody's baby wanting to get born, some other body's baby took bad sick, or something of that nature to call me away from the prayer meeting. So if I was to be at the meeting with you tonight I wouldn't never expect to stay through the prayer service.'

" 'Well, anyhow, we'll be with you in spirit when we are at the prayer meeting tonight,' they promised Aunt Jeanie.

"And then the bus was about to start. People had kept scrouging on till all the seats were filled up and folks pushed back and standing in the middle of the bus from the front to the back. Aunt Jeanie's white friend never got no seat, not being a good hand to push and shove in a crowd. And she had to stand so far up in the front that her and Aunt Jeanie couldn't even see each other to tell how they were getting along on the trip.

"After traveling long miles up the highway and stopping at every pig path to let folks get on and off, the bus came to the place where everybody had to get off that bus with all their suit satchels and things and get on other buses to go where they wanted to go. Aunt Jeanie's white friend got off and stood to one side of the bus, waiting. When Aunt Jeanie came off the bus, the colored preacher that she had sat by was helping her along, for she had taken a sick turn while she was riding on the bus.

" 'I just got a bad all-over headache,' Aunt Jeanie said to her friend, 'a bad headache with stars flashing in front of my eyes. After a little rest I'll be all right to finish this trip with you.'

"But Aunt Jeanie was bad sick and didn't know it. She started to crumple down on the sidewalk and the preacher just picked her up and carried her into the colored waiting room of the bus station. She was such a teeniny little old lady that she wasn't any load for a man to carry.

"People waiting for their buses rose up from their seats and stood back to make room for the preacher to lay Aunt Jeanie down on one of the benches. Then the preacher stayed by Aunt Jeanie to give her a cool drink and watch over the suit satchels while her friend went to find out about a place to take Aunt Jeanie where she could have doctors and be looked after to get well. It was a strange town where nobody knew Aunt Jeanie nor her white lady she was traveling with.

"The bus driver that she rode to that town with said

to her, 'Lady, you're going to miss your bus if you don't leave that old Negro woman with the other Negroes and get on your bus that's about to leave out.' But she paid him no mind.

"She found out they had a hospital in the town. Then she got a grown colored boy to help her put Aunt Jeanie in a taxi to take her to the hospital. The colored preacher had stayed to help till he nearly missed his bus. This boy was better help, for he had lived in the town for a while and knew where some places were.

"When they got to the hospital, Aunt Jeanie's friend and the colored boy started to take Aunt Jeanie inside. But the taxi driver said, 'If I was you, I'd leave her rest there on the back seat till you make the arrangements. I ain't been in this town long and I don't know whether they take colored people in this hospital or not.'

"And they didn't take colored people there. 'No,' they said to Aunt Jeanie's white friend, 'no, we can't take a sick old colored woman. No, we ain't got no place at all for Negroes here. No, we ain't never taken care of no Negroes here.'

"Some towns in this part of the country has hospitals just for colored people and some towns has places for colored people in the white folks' hospitals, and some towns don't have no hospital room for colored people at all. And this little town was the last kind.

"The white lady that brought Aunt Jeanie there argued with them and then she begged them to let her bring Aunt Jeanie into the hospital just long enough for the hospital doctors to see her and say what was the matter and not put her to bed there at all. But they said, "No. We don't treat Negroes here. And we ain't got no doctor that lives at the hospital. The doctors come from their offices in town to see the people they are waiting on in the hospital.'

"So Aunt Jeanie's friend had to think of some other place to take her. The taximan said the town didn't have no colored hotel fit for nothing. But he started back with them to help find a place. They rode by a church that was open and Aunt Jeanie's friend said, 'Stop here. At least Aunt Jeanie can lie here on a church pew and rest while the boy goes to find a doctor for her.' So they carried Aunt Jeanie inside the church and the taxi drove off.

"It was late in the day after sundown but not dark yet. The church was dim and cool for a hot August day. Big fans were whirling to cool the air. Aunt Jeanie was laid comfortable as they could make her on a wide pew at the back of the church with her friend's blue cloak folded to make a pillow. The boy said he knew the doctor that waited on his mama when she was sick and he would find him for Aunt Jeanie. So he ran to hunt up the doctor.

"The preacher of the church came in from his house next door to the church. And he said he had opened up his church and set the fans whirling to get the church ready for his Wednesday night prayer meeting. He said that inside an hour his congregation would start to come in, and he couldn't have no sick old colored woman put to bed in his church. He told the white lady to take Aunt Jeanie somewhere else.

"She said she never had no place else to take her till the doctor came. So she would have to stay in the church till then.

"Then he got mad and said he couldn't have his prayer meeting broke up in such a manner. I don't know what his words were that he said to her, but the lady said she didn't have no respect and reverence for a prayer meeting that could be broke up by a gentle old soul like Aunt Jeanie lying quiet on a back seat. And she said she aimed to stay right there and wait for the doctor. And she did that and the preacher went back to his house.

"Aunt Jeanie couldn't speak no more, but she knew enough to know that she wasn't lying in no hot, stinking colored waiting room in a bus station. And that meant a lots to her, for Aunt Jeanie was always a lady. The hatbox with the extra hats didn't work no change there. Aunt Jeanie was a lady even without a hat to her name.

"After a time the boy came hurrying in with the doctor. But he was too late to help Aunt Jeanie. One more time she had got called away from a prayer meeting place before the prayer service started. But this time it was the Almighty Himself who called her.

"The doctor was real gentle and kind and examined Aunt Jeanie careful. Then he said he couldn't have kept her from dying even if he had got there sooner, but he was sorry he couldn't get there sooner anyhow.

"The woman that played the church organ had come in and started to practice the tunes they would sing at prayer meeting. She had come in a side door and in the near-dark didn't notice the quiet folks in the back of the church. To save the confusion and fuss of an undertaker coming into the prayer meeting for Aunt Jeanie, the doctor picked her up gentle and carried her out to his car and went with her friend to take Aunt Jeanie where they would get her ready to be taken home. That night the doctor went with Aunt Jeanie's friend when she gathered up the suit satchels and the hats and the shoe box of cape jasmines and carried Aunt Jeanie back to her kin people.

"This white lady grieved deep about Aunt Jeanie dying like that away from her kin people and her not able to do nothing at all for Aunt Jeanie. But all Aunt Jeanie's friends and kin people tried to ease her grief. Jake and Hannah said to her, 'For a long time we been looking for Aunt Jeanie to be called to her long rest. And you done for her as much as her kin people could have done in her dying hour. You gave her the lovingness in your heart.'

"A lots of people that knew her came to show their respects for Aunt Jeanie. One man that was a baby she helped birth flew across the country in a silver plane to her funeral. And her church wouldn't hold half the people.

"Her colored friends, with Hannah thinking of it first, wove a blanket to cover Aunt Jeanie of smilax vines and cape jasmine flowers. They used the flowers Aunt Jeanie carried with her when she left home and people all over the country—black and white—gave their cape jasmine flowers. And it was so pretty it made the tears start in people's eyes.

"Jake and Hannah sang for Aunt Jeanie—old songs she loved best. And the colored high school choir in the county—a lots of them Aunt Jeanie's babies—sang a song called 'Lullaby at Christmas Eve.' It was the wrong reason of the year but it seemed suitable to sing the baby song for Aunt Jeanie, for she loved the solo part where the mother sings to her little baby Jesus.

"Hannah asked Mr. Sterling to read for Aunt Jeanie the same prayer that he had read at Mam Bob's funeral because Mam Bob had asked him to. It was a prayer Aunt Jeanie had read to Mam Bob from a speech by the President. Some other man had made up the prayer for the President to say, Aunt Jeanie told me when she read it to me. 'Best prayer mortal man ever left to this world,' she said to me. I ain't got a quick mind to learn things like that but I remember this much the prayer said:

" 'We are all of us children of this earth. . . . Grant us that simple knowledge. . . . Grant us a common faith that man shall know bread and peace.'

" 'Seems to me like,' Aunt Jeanie said—or was it Mam Bob?—'Seems to me like that is the nub of the whole truth on how all of us can find our race manners and keep a warm heart for people different from us and

LOURDES LIBRARY
GWYNEDD-MERCY COLLEGE
GWYNEDD VALLEY, PA 19437

people like us and make the world a good place to get born into.'

"Seems like Aunt Jeanie had that kind of warm heart for the world and the folks in it. And that brings me to the part that I have used up all these words to get to the place where I could tell you.

"Two nights ago—nearly three months since Aunt Jeanie died—Ludy sent for me to tend on her birthing. She was bad sick when I got there and punishing bad with her misery. Jake, her papa, tried his best to get a doctor for her. But it was the old story of not enough doctors in the county. Soon as he could, a doctor would come he promised. But we needed him right then.

"Never in all my years of granny-midwife work have I felt so weak and unknowing of how to get a baby into this world safe for it and the mother too. My feelings were all mixed up with praying and with wishing Aunt Jeanie was there to help. Then, like a sudden swift witness, a new strength and wisdom came into me and steadied my heart and mind and guided my hands to do the right thing. And after that Ludy birthed her baby and her and it were safe from danger. And when the doctor came he said to me, 'Aunt Jeanie herself never tended better at a birthing.'

"Then I knew what had happened to me. Aunt Jeanie *had* been there in the spirit to lend me her help and strength. Not no ghost nor no vision from heaven. I never saw anything of the kind. But for long years I have known the help and strength of Aunt Jeanie's strong and willing spirit and that was it that came to guide and strengthen me at Ludy's birthing. And knowing that, my mind picked up the last words Aunt Jeanie said to me, 'After a little rest, I'll be right back there to take hold and help out with sick folks and babies.'"

Titles in This Series

1 Charlotte Aikens, editor. *Hospital Management.* Philadelphia, 1911.

2 American Society of Superintendents of Training Schools for Nurses. *Annual Conventions*, 1893–1919.

3 John Shaw Billings and Henry M. Hurd, editors. *Hospitals, Dispensaries and Nursing: Papers and Discussion in the International Congress of Charities, Correction and Philanthropy.* Baltimore, 1894.

4 Annie M. Brainard. *The Evolution of Public Health Nursing.* Philadelphia, 1922.

5 Marie Campbell. *Folks Do Get Born.* New York, 1946.

6 *Civil War Nursing:* Louisa May Alcott. *Hospital Sketches.* Boston, 1863. *BOUND WITH Memoir of Emily Elizabeth Parsons.* Boston, 1880.

7 Committee for the Study of Nursing Education. *Nursing and Nursing Education in the United States.* New York, 1923.

8 Committee on the Grading of Nursing Schools. *Nurses, Patients and Pocketbooks.* New York, 1928.

9 Mrs. Darce Craven. *A Guide to District Nurses.* London, 1889.

10 Dorothy Deming. *The Practical Nurse.* New York, 1947.

11 Katharine J. Densford & Millard S. Everett. *Ethics for Modern Nurses.* Philadelphia, 1946.

12 Katharine D. DeWitt. *Private Duty Nursing.* Philadelphia, 1917.

13 Janet James, editor. *A Lavinia Dock Reader.*

LOURDES LIBRARY
GWYNEDD-MERCY COLLEGE
GWYNEDD VALLEY, PA 19437

14 Annette Fiske. *First Fifty Years of the Waltham Training School for Nurses*. New York, 1984. BOUND WITH Alfred Worcester. "The Shortage of Nurses—Reminiscences of Alfred Worcester '83." *Harvard Medical Alumni Bulletin 23*, 1949.

15 Virginia Henderson et al. *Nursing Studies Index, 1900–1959*. Philadelphia, 1963, 1966, 1970, 1972.

16 Darlene Clark Hine, editor. *Black Women in Nursing: An Anthology of Historical Sources*.

17 Ellen N. LaMotte. *The Tuberculosis Nurse*. New York, 1915.

18 Barbara Melosh, editor. *American Nurses in Fiction: An Anthology of Short Stories*.

19 Mary Adelaide Nutting. *A Sound Economic Basis for Schools of Nursing*. New York, 1926.

20 Sara E. Parsons. *Nursing Problems and Obligations*. Boston, 1916.

21 Juanita Redmond. *I Served on Bataan*. Philadelphia, 1943.

22 Susan Reverby, editor. *The East Harlem Health Center Demonstration: An Anthology of Pamphlets*.

23 Isabel Hampton Robb. *Educational Standards for Nurses*. Cleveland, 1907.

24 Sister M. Theophane Shoemaker. *History of Nurse-Midwifery in the United States*. Washington, D.C., 1947.

25 Isabel M. Stewart. *Education of Nurses*. New York, 1943.

26 Virginia S. Thatcher. *History of Anesthesia with Emphasis on the Nurse Specialist*. Philadelphia, 1953.

27 Adah H. Thoms. *Pathfinders—A History of the Progress of Colored Graduate Nurses*. New York, 1929.

28 Clara S. Weeks-Shaw. *A Text-Book of Nursing for the Use of Training Schools, Families, and Private Students*. New York, 1885.

29 Writers Program of the WPA in Kansas, compilers. *Lamps on the Prairie: A History of Nursing in Kansas*. Topeka, 1942.

LOURDES LIBRARY
GWYNEDD-MERCY COLLEGE
GWYNEDD VALLEY, PA 19437

LOURDES LIBRARY
GWYNEDD-MERCY COLLEGE
GWYNEDD VALLEY, PA. 19437